MOTOR DEVELOPMENT AND MOVEMENT ACTIVITIES FOR PRESCHOOLERS AND INFANTS WITH DELAYS

Second Edition

MOTOR DEVELOPMENT AND MOVEMENT ACTIVITIES FOR PRESCHOOLERS AND INFANTS WITH DELAYS

A Multisensory Approach for Professionals and Families

By

JO E. COWDEN, Ph.D.

University of New Orleans
Professor

and

CAROL C. TORREY, Ph.D.

Coordinator of Special Education Programs
Jefferson Parish Public schools

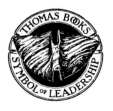

CHARLES C THOMAS • PUBLISHER, LTD.
Springfield • Illinois • U.S.A.

Published and Distributed Throughout the World by

CHARLES C THOMAS • PUBLISHER, LTD.
2600 South First Street
Springfield, Illinois 62794-9265

©2007 by CHARLES C THOMAS • PUBLISHER, LTD.

ISBN 978-0-398-07764-8 (hard)
ISBN 978-0-398-07765-5 (pbk.)

Library of Congress Catalog Card Number: 2007014825

With THOMAS BOOKS *careful attention is given to all details of manufacturing
and design. It is the Publisher's desire to present books that are satisfactory as to their
physical qualities and artistic possibilities and appropriate for their particular use.*
THOMAS BOOKS *will be true to those laws of quality that assure a good name
and good will.*

*Printed in the United States of America
MM-R-3*

Library of Congress Cataloging in Publication Data

Cowden, Jo E.
　Motor development and movement activities for preschoolers and infants
with delays : a multisensory approach for professionals and families / by
Jo E. Cowden and Carol C. Torrey. -- 2nd ed.
　　p. cm.
　Ref. ed. of: Pediatric adapted motor development and exercise. c1998.
　Includes bibliographical references and index.
　ISBN 978-0-398-07764-8 (hard) -- ISBN 978-0-398-07765-5 (pbk.)
　1. Children with disabilities--Development. 2. Exercise therapy for chil-
dren. 3. Motor ability in children. 4. Physical fitness for children. I. Torrey,
Carl C. II. Cowden, Jo E. Pediatric adapted motor development and exer-
cise. III. Title.

RJ138.C68 2007
615.8'2083--dc22   2007014825

PREFACE

The second edition of the book is intended to provide information for professionals, families, and students interested in learning about motor development of young children with delays or disabilities. A practical approach is used so that families and caregivers can provide instruction utilizing the ecological dynamics of the home environment. The book emphasizes the age group of infancy (6 months) to 6 years. However, families with older children and professionals who work with older children who have significant motor delays will also benefit from the information and activities in this book. Activities are specifically designed for parents of children with delays/disabilities and specialists of motor development, adapted physical education, special education, early childhood, early intervention and allied health.

The purpose of the book is to explain the principles of motor developmental theories and relate them to practical intervention, answer questions about muscle tone (hypotonicity, hypertonicity) related to positioning, lifting, carrying, and feeding of young children, provide directions for early diagnosis and assessment of symptoms recognizable in developmental domains including autism, and help professionals and families understand the impact of medical conditions on motor development and related daily living skills for young children. In addition, practical suggestions and activities for families and professionals to enhance sensory motor development of the young child during structured motor intervention and throughout the day are provided.

Throughout this book, the term "movement specialist" has been used to refer to one of the many professionals that provide motor assessment and activities to young children with disabilities. This array of professionals may include, but is not limited to: adapted physical educator, occupational therapist, physical therapist, early childhood educator, preschool classroom teacher, home-based early intervention teacher, and so forth. Regardless of the title of this professional, a movement specialist will have been trained in the psychomotor domain, and will have knowledge to provide appropriate and valuable motor assessment and intervention to young children with disabilities. Additionally, it must be noted that a para-educator (teacher assistant) may also be provided specific training to complete intervention.

JO E. COWDEN
CAROL C. TORREY

ACKNOWLEDGMENTS

The authors wish to acknowledge: Connie L. Phelps, Chair of Reference Services Earl K. Long Library at the University of New Orleans who provided detailed assistance for the references in this book.

The families and children with delays or disabilities who have participated in motor interventions during the past 25 years at The University of New Orleans, and who have provided us learning and expertise in the field of motor interventions.

Jean Burke, whose friendship, faith, humor, and love have provided me with the wisdom necessary for completion of this revision.

Margaret Huffman, Jo's sister, who has provided love, faith, and incredible strength.

Peter Torrey, and my two daughters, Alexandra and Alanna Torrey, for their patience, encouragement, and love while I worked endlessly on the revision of this book.

Our friend, Anita Hartzell Hefler, who administers the program at the Greater New Orleans Therapeutic Riding Center, encouraging excellence in the young children with disabilities and working with university students in adapted physical education practices.

I also want to dedicate this publication to the memory of my beloved pup, Chelsea Makala Cowden, who stayed very close to her mom for 15 years providing companionship for hours of writing.

Michael Payne Thomas and Claire Slagle of Charles C Thomas Publisher who provided incredible leadership and support for developing this book.

JEC
CCT

CONTENTS

MOTOR DEVELOPMENT AND MOVEMENT ACTIVITIES FOR PRESCHOOLERS AND INFANTS WITH DELAYS

Chapter 1

MOTOR DEVELOPMENT

Chapter Objectives: After studying this chapter, the reader will be able to:
1. Relate the importance of the interaction between the child and environment;
2. Give a meaningful definition of motor development;
3. Explain the principles of Motor Development Theory;
4. Provide a summary of traditional developmental theories, neurodevelopmental theories and Dynamic Systems Theory (DST).

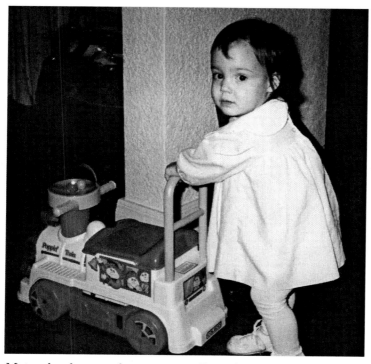

Figure 1.1. Motor development begins prenatally and continues throughout the lifespan as repetitive practice and increasingly difficult challenges expand one's motor skills.

3

INTERACTION OF CHILD AND THE ENVIRONMENT

The interaction of a young child with his/her environment provides critical opportunities for motor development, as well as development within all of the other learning domains (language, self-help, cognitive, social). The interplay between forces within the individual and the environment is referred to by Gallahue and Ozmun (2006) as *adaptation,* while Sherrill (2004) referred to changes within the individual, the environment and the blend of both the individual and everything in his environment as *ecological theory.* Most professionals agree that the child's environment is critical in the learning process and that valuable opportunities for learning experiences are provided through interaction with an enriched environment. Thus, the importance of early intervention is highlighted.

An understanding of motor development theory and principles of normal motor development influence one's ability to administer motor assessments and to develop motor intervention programs for young children with delays or abnormal motor development. The needs of young children place specific challenges on movement specialists or teachers who provide service delivery in the motor domain. A unique understanding of varied theoretical perspectives, combined with the talents of selecting the appropriate plan of action result in development of optimal movement programs. Philosophical concepts are applied and incorporated into performance objectives for intervention and provide the framework or structure for long-term goals or outcomes. Combining elements from the various traditional, neurodevelopmental, and contemporary theories is the key to successful individualization of intervention curricula for preschoolers and infants with delays. An overview of selected theoretical perspectives will be briefly discussed within this theoretical framework.

A theoretical basis of motor development provides a basis for linking assessment and intervention processes. A theoretical background assists the movement specialist in understanding the relationship between normal and abnormal motor development. Each movement specialist who participates in the evaluation process develops an internal schema that depicts mature versus immature patterns of movement. A critical reference is then needed to determine if the immature patterns actually have a neurological orientation that would indicate possible central nervous system damage associated with abnormal motor developmental patterns (e.g., cerebral palsy). The specialist establishes an assessment approach based on his or her theoretical frame of reference. The following model (see Figure 1.2) will assist in clarifying the link between theory, assessment, and intervention. Theories included in this model are summarized following the model.

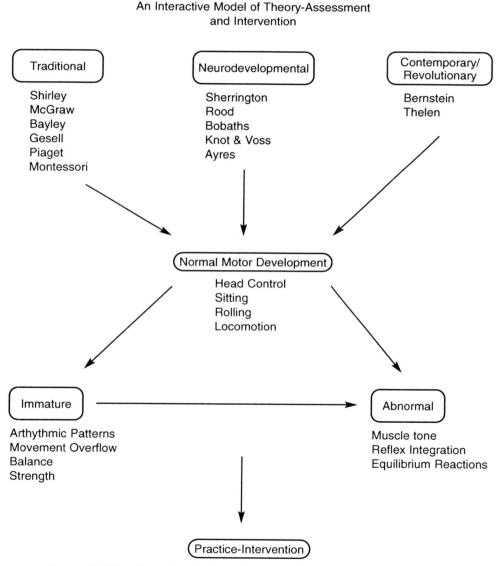

Figure 1.2. The Model for Linking Theory, Assessment, and Intervention.

MOTOR DEVELOPMENT THEORIES

Prior to discussing the various motor development theories, it is important to define some terms related to early childhood development. **Motor development** may be defined as changes of movement behavior across the lifespan including growth, development, and maturation. The process of motor development is continuous and age-related and includes growth, maturation, and development. **Growth** involves quantitative biological and structural changes of the physical size of the child. **Maturation** is defined as qualitative changes that occur as a function of time and age. **Development** includes functional changes which lead to compensation by the individual throughout the lifespan. There is a fixed and sequential order of development; however, rate of change may vary (Gallahue & Ozmun, 2006; Malina, 1975; Payne & Isaacs, 2005; Seefelt, 1989; Sherrill, 2004).

Traditional Developmental Theories

Traditional developmental theories are based on a hierarchical model of motor skill acquisition. Shirley (1931) proposed a neuromaturational theory of motor development that suggested interindividual variability exists in the motor development of young children. Shirley (1931) outlined five specific phases of motor development: "(a) development of passive postural control; (b) development of active postural control; (c) active efforts toward locomotion; (d) locomotion by creeping and walking with support, and (e) walking alone" (p. 193). These phases develop sequentially and can be correlated with observational assessment of infant movement and play.

McGraw (1932, 1940, 1945) analyzed the development of motor patterns in relation to functional growth and maturation of the nervous system. She emphasized that developmental phases must be carefully studied and understood to increase practical value of standardized tests. McGraw recorded observations of infant behavior in prone progression including neonatal swimming actions, suspended inversion and postural adjustment, rolling, sitting, erect posture, and upright locomotion. She concluded that reflexive movements appear prior to controlled motor patterns and that maturation influences acquisition of upright locomotion. New motor patterns emerge gradually, although stress may increase the use of immature patterns. Her diagrams of erect locomotion are continually used in efforts to better understand infant development.

During this time period, Bayley (1936) developed one of the first motor scales to objectively quantify infant motor development. Her longitudinal study of mental and motor development remains one of the most intricate and complex of human development studies. The *Bayley Scales on Infant Development* is one of the more widely-used standardized instruments in clinical settings (Fewell & Glick, 1996), and it is projected that the newest edition of the instrument, *The Bayley Scales of Infant and Toddler Development, Third Edition* (2006) will continue to provide valuable assessment information.

Gesell (1928, 1939, 1949, 1954) suggested the following principles of motor development: (a) development is governed by maturation, (b) development occurs in cephalocaudal and proximodistal directions, (c) development occurs asymmetrically, and (d) progression within various developmental domains occurs at uneven paces. Gesell emphasized an intermesh or a spiraling view of development resulting in a complex model of dynamic behavior. He also suggested that an infant's upright postural stability is dependent on the process of reciprocal innervation, whether reflexive or voluntary, and progressive reintegration of muscle groups is prerequisite to subsequent motor development. Many of these principles continue to guide assessment processes and standardized testing (Sherrill, 2004) (see Figure 1.3).

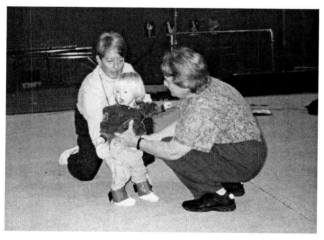

Figure 1.3. The movement specialist and physical therapist collaborate to assess the strength and balance of an infant with Down syndrome.

Additionally, Piaget (1952, 1985) highlighted the importance of the environment and active involvement in the environment as critical to child development. He emphasized the following: (a) continuous development occurs in a fixed and defined order through four sequential stages (i.e., sensorimotor period, preoperational period, concrete operations, formal operations); (b) there are individual differences in rate of development; and (c) through self-organization, sensorimotor experiences influence the quality of cognitive processes. Piagetian principles are utilized throughout early intervention and link assessment to programming strategies.

Montessori, an Italian physician who began her work with children with disabilities, developed the Montessori Method which was based, in part, on the efforts of Itard and Sequin in associationistic psychology (DeVries & Kohlberg, 1990; Moran & Kalakian, 1974). Montessori was the original proponent of "sensorial education" through activities which involve both intelligence and movement (Montessori, 1936a/1956, 1936b/1966, 1949/1967). The Montessori Method allows the child the freedom to interact independently in a prepared environment that is filled with age-appropriate child-size furnishings and toys. The environment is arranged systematically to promote the child's progressive interests and personality development (Montessori, 1909/1964, 1914/1965). Exercises in daily living, sensory materials, and conceptual elements promote the child's construction of independence, self-control, self-reliance, and intrinsic rewards. Montessori recognized the connection between mental and motor development, "But to always be thinking of the mind, on the one hand, and the body, on the other, is to break the continuity that should reign between them" (1967, p. 171). Thus, there is a cyclic relationship between mental and motor development whereby one promotes the other and the working of the mind and body elevates the child to higher learning planes.

Neurodevelopmental Theories

Sherrington (1906) originated the reflex model of motor control which influenced many subsequent theories. His principles of normal motor development were utilized to better understand problems of abnormal motor development and central nervous system dysfunction. The term proprioception was derived by Sherrington (1906) to refer to the perception of sensation as initiating in the sensory receptors and stimulated by an organism's own movement. The nervous system is the interactive component for which no part is capable of reaction without affecting another part and is never completely at rest.

Rood (1956) developed a neurophysiological theory for remediation of sensorimotor delays that states motor functions are inseparable from sensory system components. As indicated in Sherrill (1993), Rood's model of mobility-stability includes motor progression from a pattern of total flexion to independent walking. Rolling, prone-lying with hyperextension of the entire spine, prone-lying with contraction of neck muscles, prone-lying with weight on elbows, kneeling on hands and knees, and standing are intermediate steps. In accord with this theory, motor activities should be completed along with sensory stimulation, including techniques such as icing, brushing, and deep muscle pressure.

Bobath and Bobath (1964) originated the neurodevelopmental theory, a philosophy of treatment for the neurological disorder of cerebral palsy. The Bobaths' theory emphasized that normal development results from the proper integration of reflexes and the emergence of postural reactions. This theory promoted the development of what the Bobaths termed the "normal postural reflex mechanism." Based on their theoretical premises, normal development results from the proper integration of reflexes and the emergence of postural reactions.

Knott and Voss (1968) referred to the proprioceptive neuromuscular facilitation (PNF) method which is based on principles of normal motor development and motor learning, initial assessment of performance level, and individualized treatment. Four features of PNF are: (a) stimulation of proprioceptors, (b) training of coordination by combinations of movement patterns, (c) use of maximal and adjusted resistance to promote initiation of movement patterns, and (d) specific movement techniques (Knott & Voss, 1968).

Ayres (1972, 1974, 1980, 1989) originated a neurobehavioral theory of sensory integration which suggested that input into the central nervous system begins at the lowest level and proceeds to each successive level. Movement therapy should therefore be directed to six different levels within the central nervous system: (a) spinal cord, (b) brain stem, (c) cerebellum, (d) basal ganglia, (e) limbic system, and (f) cortex. Therapy should involve: (a) the relationship of brain anatomy and motor functioning, (b) tactile stimulation, (c) swinging and spinning activities for vestibular stimulation, (d) activities involving extensor

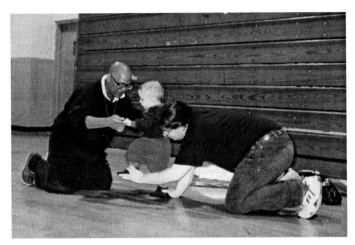

Figure 1.4. The movement specialist provides direction to the father of a young child with developmental delay to facilitate a walking pattern.

muscles, and (e) body control activities. The process of motor learning and development can also be understood through the "Spiraling Continuum Adaptation Theory" (Gilfoyle, Grady, & Moore, 1981). The spiraling process emphasizes the interaction of sensory input, motor output, and sensory feedback and emphasizes three important principles: (1) a child's adaptation to new experiences is dependent on past acquired behaviors, (2) new experiences are integrated with past experiences so that past behaviors are modified and result in higher level behavior, and (3) higher level behaviors influence and increase the maturity of the lower level behaviors. Through the adaptation process, children acquire purposeful behaviors and actions which become skilled performance.

Principles of Motor Development Theories

This section provides suggested principles of motor development in accord with traditional developmental and neurodevelopmental theories that assist individuals with a basic understanding of the motor systems of infants and young children. These principles may not be prerequisites of thought for all theoretical foundations, but they provide a beginning structure for developing the premises necessary to implement motor intervention programs for young children. Table 1.1 provides a list of the principles of motor development.

Table 1.1 Principles of Motor Development.

1. Maturation of the nervous system
2. Cephalocaudal and proximodistal development
3. Reflex integration
4. Equilibrium reactions matured
5. General to specific movements
6. Intersensory integration activated
7. Motor output organized
8. Functional postural integration

Principle 1: Maturation of the Nervous System

The extent of the maturity of the nervous system is based on the degree of neuronal myelination. **Myelination** is the process of forming a white protein insulation covering of nerve fiber pathways within the central nervous system (CNS). The myelin sheath preserves energy and maintains speed of nerve impulse conduction. CNS tracts become myelinated in a definite order and according to an inherently determined process. The degree to which myelination has been completed is an indicator of functional sensorimotor pathways, thus, an indicator of manual and locomotor skill development. The somesthetic (tactile-kinesthetic) system is the first of the sensory modalities to begin the process of myelination at approximately the eighth prenatal month followed by the vestibular, visual and auditory systems (Espenschade & Eckert, 1980; Sherrill, 1981; Williams, 1983).

Espenschade and Eckert (1980) summarized changes that occur after birth in the degree of myelination of the nervous system and the resulting motoric action. The principle of cephalocaudal and proximodistal directions heavily influences the major motor milestones accomplished after the myelination process has occurred to specific parts of the CNS. For example, around 12 months of age the pyramidal tracts are heavily myelinated and the resulting motor skill development includes standing and walking alone as well as manual development of the pincer grasp and release of objects. Complexity of movements following myelination of the cerebellum is demonstrated by the development of one-foot hopping and alternate foot stair-climbing. Myelination of the corpus callosum is a predictor of the immediate development of optimal alternate arm-leg action in such activities as throwing and kicking (see Figure 1.5). The corpus callosum joins the two hemispheres of the cerebrum and permits exchange of informa-

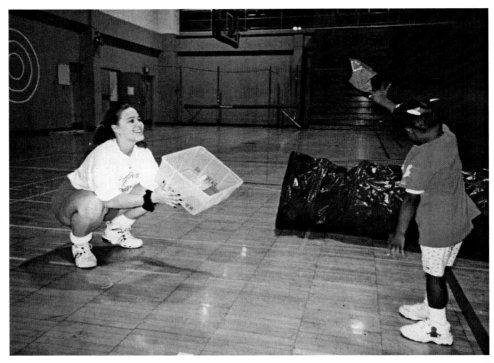

Figure 1.5. Alternate arm-leg throwing is a complex skill which follows myelination of the corpus callosum, has not yet been attained by this preschool child.

tion between the right and left brain hemispheres, thus facilitating the alternating, oppositional arm and leg patterns.

Principle 2: Cephalocaudal and Proximodistal Development

Growth and maturation of the infant proceeds according to specific developmental directions. **Cephalocaudal development** in the human being occurs from the head downward to the feet. The child's head is much larger at birth in proportion to the rest of the body. Therefore, movement patterns must first be developed in the muscles of the upper body to provide stabilization of the head, neck, and trunk (see Figure 1.6). Cephalocaudal development is clearly illustrated by Dunn and Leitschuh (2006). At birth, the infant is in a prone position, then moves through various lateral postures, and ultimately transitions to upright posture, whereby the young child then has the skill to move in varied locomotor patterns.

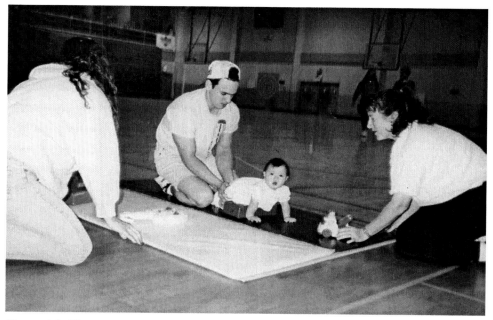

Figure 1.6. The movement specialist is addressing optimum prone positioning with the father of an infant with Down syndrome.

This principle is especially important in relation to assessment. Early reflex and voluntary movements are dependent upon directional movements of the head and the strength of the neck muscles. As trunk development increases in strength, leg movements are generated primarily from power initiated by the hip flexors. Several motor theories suggest that spiraling, nonlinear, multimodal system approaches provide explanations that offer more clarity to sensory and motor interrelationships than the specific principle of cephalocaudal and proximodistal development (Gesell, 1939; Gilfoyle et al., 1981; Knott & Voss, 1968; Thelen, 1995). *However, beyond any doubt, the head plays a major role in the performance of typical motor skills and the movement of the head initiates primitive reflex patterns.*

Proximodistal development means that muscular movements near the midline of the body become more refined before those more distal from the midline. For example, the child will grasp and bring objects to the mouth before he or she will reach out extending the elbow, arm, and fingers to pick-up a peg and place it into a pegboard. Catching or trapping a ball at the center of the trunk of the body would precede extension of the arm and hand away from the midline of the body to catch a tossed object (Cratty, 1979; Eichstaedt & Kalakian, 1993; Espenschade & Eckert, 1980; & Sherrill, 1998).

Principle 3: Reflex Integration

Primitive reflexes are typical, involuntary movements that must be inhibited or integrated by the CNS. These reflexes provide repetitive flexion and extension movements during the first 4 months of infant development and purposefully assist the infant with exploration of his or her environment. However, after this time period the primitive reflexes will become integrated. The presence of primitive reflexes beyond 6–8 months of age may interfere with the child obtaining functional mobility skills. For example, the tonic neck group of reflexes (asymmetrical and symmetrical tonic neck reflexes and the tonic labyrinthine prone and supine reflexes) must be suppressed before the child can learn to roll, crawl, and creep (Fiorentino, 1963; Holle, 1981; Milani-Comparetti, 1987; Milani-Comparetti & Gidoni, 1967; Sherrill, 2004). Figure 1.7 illustrates the need for reflex integration as a young child crawls forward reaching for a toy. Retention of primitive reflex patterns may also cause young children to lack rhythmical interaction and efficiency of movement which appears through observation as poor equilibrium and balance, lack of postural integration, and poor visual motor coordination.

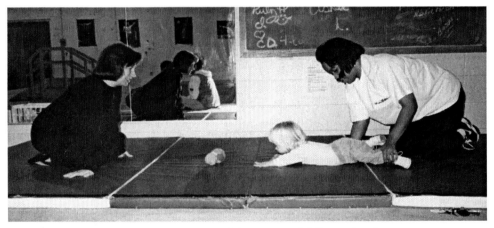

Figure 1.7. The interventionist gives guidelines to a child's mother for increasing extensor tone and proximodistal reach.

Principle 4: Equilibrium Reactions Matured

Reactions (righting, equilibrium, and parachute) are automatic movements that replace the primitive reflexes with unique functions necessary for the development of balance. **Righting reactions** assist with the alignment of the head and trunk with each other. For example, rotation of the head and neck causes the rest of the body to roll over in the same direction. **Parachute reactions** are protective extension movements which occur when the child starts to fall or lose his balance. **Equilibrium or tilting reactions** are compensatory movements which allow the child to adjust posture and maintain stability while in the prone, supine, sitting, quadruped or standing positions (see Figure 1.8) (Dunn & Leitschuh, 2006; Gilfoyle et al., 1981; Holle, 1981; Parks, 2006; Sherrill, 2004).

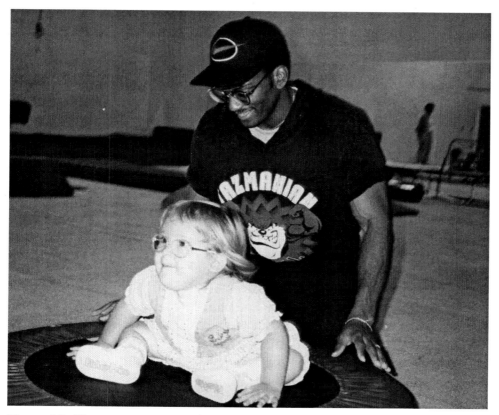

Figure 1.8. The movement specialist is providing an activity to develop equilibrium responses in a young child with spina bifida.

Principle 5: General to Specific Movements

The child will develop movements of the large muscle groups of the trunk before developing specific movements of the extremities (arms, legs, fingers, and feet). Random or reflexive movements may be observed in the extremities; however, the movements are without intentional purpose on the part of the infant (e.g., kicking and flexion and extensor thrusting action of legs). Creeping provides an example of a specific process of development from general to specific movements. Key behaviors associated with creeping involve postural strategies of the trunk against gravity (head lift, prone extension, and hand-knee position) combined with reciprocal limb actions to move the body in space. Another example of general to specific development is sitting. As balance is achieved in the sitting position, one and then both hands are freed simultaneously for eye-hand coordination activities (Eichstaedt & Kalakian, 1993; Gilfoyle et al., 1981; Sherrill, 2004) (see Figure 1.9).

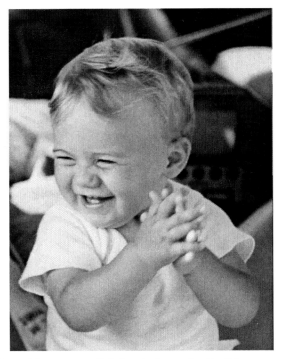

Figure 1.9. With the achievement of sitting independently this young child will be able to refine a more specific eye-hand coordination skill of clapping with hands in midline.

Principle 6: Intersensory Integration Activated

The young child is constantly bombarded with sensory input from the tactile, kinesthetic, vestibular, visual, and auditory systems. However, many infants, toddlers, and preschoolers with developmental delays experience problems with **intersensory integration** or the ability to use simultaneous input from several modalities. The child exhibits constant changes in muscle tone due to sensory input indicating that intersensory modality input is not yet integrated or nerve pathways have not matured. Fine tuning or the development of smooth, efficient movements comes through repeated cycles of action while modifying their current movement dynamics. Williams (1983) stated,

> There is little doubt that we do learn to integrate sensory information—that we come to recognize what kinds of sounds accompany a talking face or how an object that moves or has certain characteristics actually feels. This process is believed to involve the gradual integration by the child (through countless experiences) of all available stimulus information surrounding a given environmental event into one complex sensory matrix or picture. (p. 144)

Therefore, it is imperative that sensory strengths and weaknesses are determined when possible and specific sensory stimulation exercises and activities that allow for intersensory exploration are provided (Sherrill, 2004; Williams, 1983) (see Figure 1.10).

Principle 7: Motor Output Organized

Motor output must be evaluated to determine the abilities or degree of developmental delay in a young child. According to Sherrill (1993), motor behaviors or actions may appear as three types of movements: (a) reflex, (b) reaction or automatic response, and (c) skill. In general, to remediate delays, exercises should be programmed that suppress or inhibit primitive reflex patterns and promote equilibrium reactions which will assist in the development of coordinated or skilled movements. Therefore, experiences that help young children organize motor outputs must be provided.

During the sensorimotor period of development (birth to age 2), specific motor outputs that should be evaluated include reflex analysis, emergence of equilibrium reactions and balance, muscle tone reaction to movements, mobility and stability, postural or bilateral integration, prehension skills and voluntary release, visual responses and

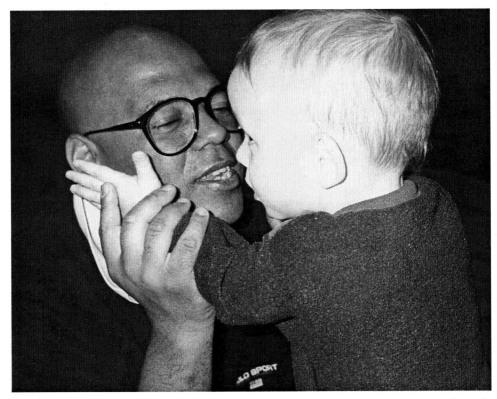

Figure 1.10. The movement specialist is encouraging intersensory integration through tactile and auditory modalities with a child who has a visual impairment.

tracking abilities, and tactile sensitivity (Cowden & Torrey, 1995). After age two, perceptual-motor functions that should also be assessed include fundamental motor skills (running, jumping, hopping, skipping, climbing stairs, kicking, and catching/throwing), physical and motor fitness (muscular strength, endurance, flexibility, cardiovascular endurance, balance, agility, speed, coordination, and reaction time), motor planning/sequencing, and imitation of movements (Cowden & Torrey, 1995; Cratty, 1964; Sherrill, 1993) (see Figure 1.11).

Principle 8: Functional Postural Integration

Children should learn to coordinate **bilateral movements** (both sides of the body or the upper and lower parts of the body), **unilateral movements** (one side of the body, e.g., right arm and right leg moving simultaneously), and **crosslateral** or **midline crossing**

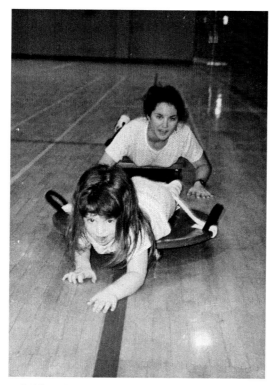

Figure 1.11. A young child with spina bifida is encouraged to increase her upper body strength and organize her motor output during a scooterboard activity.

movements (right arm and left leg or left leg and right arm). Young children with multisystem delays often demonstrate associated reactions in which they are unable to perform movements on one side of the body without "overflow" of movements to the other side of the body. Gesell (1949) included the development of functional asymmetrical movements or the development of a preferred side of the body as a principle of maturation. Several early neurodevelopmentalists (Gesell, 1939; Knott & Voss, 1968; Rood, 1954, 1956) stressed the importance of establishing a process of interweaving and reciprocal relationships of antagonistic functions of muscle groups to develop efficient postural integration. Postural integration is often an area of difficulty experienced by young children and requires critical and sensitive observational assessment to determine appropriate intervention activities.

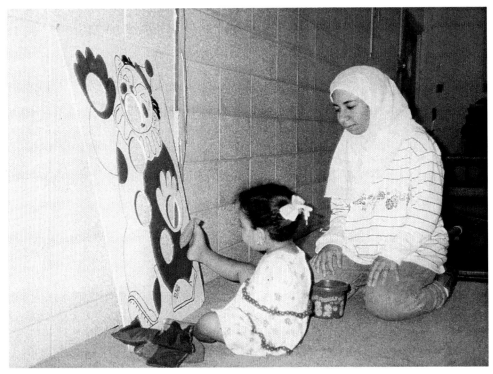

Figure 1.12. This child makes use of her feet during beanbag play due to her congenital birth defect.

CONTEMPORARY DYNAMIC SYSTEMS THEORY

Contemporary Dynamic Systems Theory (DST) models of early motor development have emerged which challenge the traditional basis of motor development and provide new concepts for understanding total action systems and motor development of infants and young children (Kelso, 1982; Thelen, Kelso, & Fogel, 1987; Thelen & Smith, 1994; Thelen & Ulrich, 1991). A more in-depth review of the model will be examined as, "Dynamic Systems Theory postulates that new forms of behavior emerge from the cooperative interactions of multiple components within a task context" (Thelen & Ulrich, 1991, p. v). This approach provides alternatives for uncovering the processes that young children with delays may utilize to acquire motor skills.

DST provides a theoretical philosophy which may serve as a bridge between motor control and motor development. The theory offers a contemporary explanation of how movement is initiated, how it is controlled, and how changes occur throughout the developmental process. Thus, the process becomes the focus (Thelen, 1989). Crutchfield and Barnes (1993) stated, "According to dynamic action theory, movement is not prescribed, but emerges in relation to the external environment and the internal biologic environment" (p. 42). Throughout the literature, several terms are being used interchangeably, such as dynamic action systems, systems theory, dynamic pattern generation, dynamical systems approach, and dynamic motor theory. The emerging discipline as it relates to motor development in the behavioral and neurosciences and the field of biomechanics has been referred to by Lockman and Thelen (1993) as "developmental biodynamics."

Prior to the formulation of DST, traditional developmental theories (Gessel, 1939, 1946; Gessell & Ames, 1940; McGraw, 1932, 1940, 1946) proposed that development was a linear, stage-like progression of increasingly more functional, sequential behaviors. This progression toward adult forms of behavior proceeds according to a grand plan that is scheduled by a grand timekeeper (Thelen & Smith, 1994). Each of these traditional theories represented the cerebral cortex as a diverse and purposeful organ. As maturity progresses, all neuromuscular systems responsible for active and purposeful movement increasingly take over control. This self-organizing pattern of specific neuromuscular actions that reflect dynamic movements are beliefs held in common with DST and the early developmentalists (Thelen & Bates, 2003).

DST and its relationship to concepts of Piagetian (1951, 1952) philosophy allow for a range of individual differences through the process of variability. Children may learn new information in different manners, but with similar outcomes. Especially important is the similarity between DST and the work of Piaget in emphasis on the interaction of the environment and the organism. However, Piaget's (1985) theoretical concepts of developmental change relating to cognitive development during the sensorimotor period of an infant are in conflict with DST. DST theorists suggest the human infant is highly competent and capable of more than reflexive responses to external stimuli and possesses "highly structured perceptual and conceptual skills" (Thelen & Smith, 1994, p. 22).

Thelen has collaborated with numerous researchers to study the application and interpretation of DST to the motor development of young children. Thelen and Fisher (1982, 1983a, 1983b; Thelen, Fisher, & Ridley-Johnson, 1984) examined infants' movements (i.e., supine kicking and the disappearing stepping reflex) to gain a better understanding of how infants were learning movement patterns which they proposed were unaccounted for by traditional motor development and neural maturational theories. They further provided this explanation for the disappearance of the stepping reflex: "infants legs simply grew heavy with subcutaneous fat, making it impossible to lift them when infants were supported upright" (Thelen & Bates, 2003, p. 380). Additionally Galloway and Thelen (2003) noted that infants gain control of their feet prior to control of their hands, thus questioning the traditional principal of cephalocaudal development (see Figure 1.12).

Thelen refined the 6 components (see Table 1.2) as they apply to locomotor coordination during the first year of life, thus providing a perspective of skill acquisition (e.g., Thelen, 1983, 1985, 1989; Thelen & Cooke, 1987; Thelen & Fogel, 1989; Thelen, et. al., 1987; Thelen, Ulrich, & Jensen, 1989). In more recent studies (1992, 1994, 1995) she provided new insights into the process by which infants and young

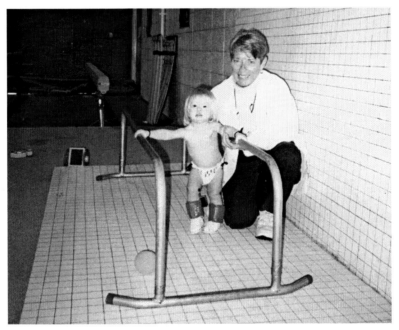

Figure 1.13. Passive and active contributing subsystems are facilitated by cooperative interactions between the child and interventionist.

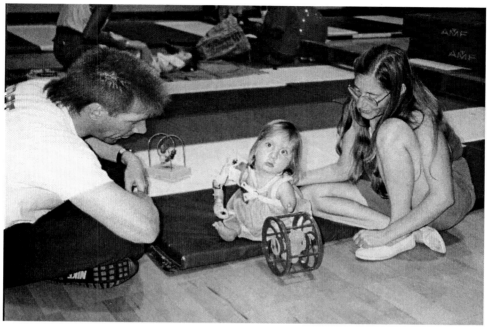

Figure 1.14. The contributing subsystems and anatomical constraints of a young child with multiple congenital anomalies must be determined prior to developing a sequence of intervention goals and activities.

children learn movement control. Adopting the contributions of Bernstein (1967), Thelen's theoretical application of DST relates movement to cooperative interactive processes, internal and external organizational stability, and environmental contributions. Bernstein proposed the concept of "degrees of freedom" of movement for each joint. Controlling for all the possible combinations of movements by neurons, muscles and joints becomes an overwhelming complex problem of the central nervous system. New patterns of movement become preferred patterns only under certain conditions. If all the internal and external conditions are not met, the organism will undergo many behavioral changes to seek stability and bring order to a disorganized system (Thelen, 1989; Thelen & Ulrich, 1991). To suggest application of DST to children with delays or disabilities, other contributing factors might include type of disability, age, growth, anatomical constraints, postural control mechanisms, skeleton-muscular apparatus, motivational status, environmental contexts, and instructions for the task (see Figure 1.13).

Components of Dynamic Systems Theory

This section highlights the components of DST which are most often applied to movement of infants and young children. The components are presented in a sequential order according to the authors' interpretation of the relationship among the components. Table 1.2 summarizes the components of DST.

Table 1.2. Components of Dynamic Systems Theory

1. The brain is a self-organizing system
2. Degrees of freedom and collective variables or coordinative structures
3. Attractor states
4. Phase shifts
5. Control parameters
6. Rate limiters

Component 1: The Brain is a Self-Organizing System

Dynamic systems theorists view the brain as a "dynamic and self organizing system" versus a "hard-wired and static structure" (Thelen, 1987, p. 13), and acknowledge that the physical and social environments are equal contributors with neural maturation (Thelen & Fogel, 1989). Due to the complex and dynamic nature of all the contributing components, the developmental process is asynchronous, asymmetrical, and nonlinear in developmental and real time (Thelen, 1987, 1989). Motor development is interpreted as a learning process which combines the child's existing abilities with new task requirements and constraints. New patterns will develop that can later be generalized to subsequent novel but similar situations (Thelen, 1994).

Based on the movement pattern that results from the **contributing subsystems**, there may be differences in individual sequences of development, due to the child's system's abilities to self-organize the variables from the contributing subsystems. (see Figure 1.14). Children with the same diagnosis may achieve developmental milestones in a different order and rate, and with very different movement patterns. Each developmental task must therefore be analyzed in relation to the particular environmental context and may require a task analysis approach (Thelen, 1989; Thelen & Ulrich, 1991).

DST gives equal consideration to neurological, genetic, and environmental constraints. When efficiency of movement and functioning is a goal for the child with a delay or disability, it may not always be appropriate to allow the child's motor system to self-organize. The self-organization may lead to atypical or inefficient patterns. In many situations, knowledge of all medical complications and the site of CNS damage guides the intervention.

Component 2: Degrees of Freedom and Collective Variables or Coordinative Structures

As previously discussed, Bernstein (1967) describes "degrees of freedom" for the movement of each joint (e.g., flexion, abduction, and rotation). DST suggests an individual's systems self-organize these degrees of freedom, reducing them from an almost limitless combination of muscles, joints, and neuronal elements into a more concise and stable form of movement. The combinations of elements that are expressed in the development of new movement forms are referred to as **collective variables or coordinative structures** (Thelen & Fogel, 1989; Thelen, 1989). These collective variables have spatial and temporal precision.

One might conceptualize that a child with Down syndrome may have additional degrees of freedom at a joint. The presence of hypotonicity and joint laxity add variability to the child's movement patterns. The absence of neurological damage may allow the child to compress degrees of freedom in a unique manner, such as locking knees for greater stability during creeping (see Figure 1.15) or utilizing excessive joint laxity (abduction and outward rotation) in the hip to scoot forward on her buttocks. Also, as the child begins to acquire independent walking skills, she may exhibit an unusually wide base of support with arms in an exaggerated high guard position and knee locking in order to stabilize upright locomotor posture. During step initiation, the forward swing of her lower limbs may begin with external rotation causing a waddling gait pattern.

Component 3: Attractor States

The new collective variables or coordinative structures may become the child's preferred patterns of movement under certain conditions. These new patterns of movement are referred to as **attractor states** (Thelen & Fogel, 1989; Thelen, 1989). The child's system prefers to

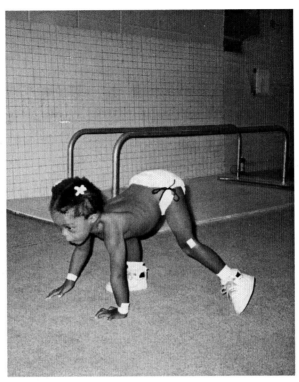

Figure 1.15. Self-organization by this child's CNS leads to the "locking of joints" to gain stability, a pattern of movement that interferes with typical upright locomotion.

work from this attractor state but may also choose other options as the behavior is still free to fluctuate within the preferred limits of the degrees of freedom (Thelen, 1992).

The young child with a delay or disability may utilize abnormal or atypical patterns when moving independently (e.g., a child with Down syndrome creeping with knees locked). These patterns may be a result of neurological or muscular damage or anatomical features of the disability (e.g., joint laxity). Through individualized intervention programs, the child may gradually learn to use more efficient patterns (e.g., creeping with the knees touching the floor) (see Figure 1.16).

Component 4: Phase Shifts

If all of the internal and external conditions for this attractor state (preferred pattern of movement) are not met, the child's system may undergo vast behavioral changes known as **phase shifts** (Thelen,

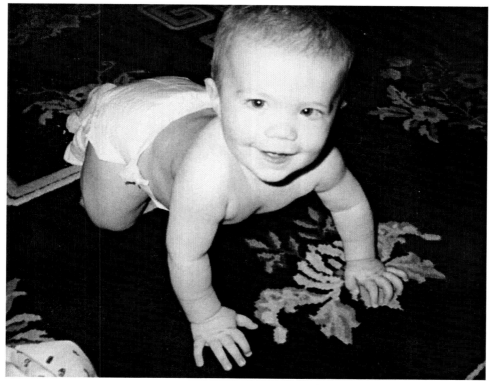

Figure 1.16. A typical creeping patterns with the knees touching the floor requires flexion and extension of the hips and knees, a precursor to stepping.

1985, 1989; Thelen & Ulrich, 1991). During a phase shift, the central and peripheral nervous systems search for a new level of stability based on history, social and physical environment, and the individual's intentions (Thelen, 1983, 1989, 1995). The child's system transitions between two attractor states; however, this transition may be less stable than either of the two original attractor states.

For a child with cerebral palsy (Kamm, Thelen, & Jensen, 1990), the typical developmental pattern of symmetrical kicking is often not the preferred pattern of movement (the attractor state). Due to damage of the central nervous system, dissociation of the lower extremities from the upper extremities and the lack of coordination between the central and peripheral nervous system occurs. The movement pattern lacks smooth, coordinated symmetrical kicking: legs may be rigid and stiff, or flaccid and hypotonic. In addition to central nervous system dysfunction, a young child with cerebral palsy may be affected by numerous subsystems such as arousal, posture, and task constraints. The environment and interaction with others must be modified to provide a balance of relaxation and stimulation for efficient movement.

Component 5: Control Parameters

While the child's system is searching for stability during a phase shift, the system may be sensitive to changes in particular internal or external variables. These variables are referred to as **control parameters** and can cause reorganization of the entire system (Thelen, 1989). Control parameters do not control the system, prescribe change, or represent change; however, they move the system through various preferred patterns of movement (attractor states) (Thelen, 1989; Thelen & Ulrich, 1991).

For a child with cerebral palsy, prior to or during periods of transition from one position to another or during the acquisition of a higher level skill, the child may need a caregiver to intervene with guided facilitation of movement patterns (see Figure 1.17). The child may exhibit hypertonicity and delayed reflex integration. Through proper positioning and handling techniques, the child may gradually learn to mobilize or maintain a position without the interference of delayed reflexes. However, if the child is not properly relaxed and positioned, he may not have the opportunity to function within the preferred attractor state. He may be limited to the degrees of freedom he can compress into an atypical or abnormal movement pattern that helps him achieve his purpose for movement.

Component 6: Rate Limiters

There may be different rates of development among the six components of DST: development is asynchronous and asymmetrical. The slowest developing component is **rate limiting** (Thelen, 1989), whereby the slowest developing component affects how well the individual can exhibit a movement pattern. Any of the contributing subsystems (e.g., anatomical constraints, task instructions, maturation, postural stability, motivation etc.) may be a potential rate-limiter in a given context. This rate-limiting variable is often also the control parameter (Thelen & Ulrich, 1991).

DST allows the movement specialist to intervene with prepared strategies or exercises to guide development of muscle tone, strength

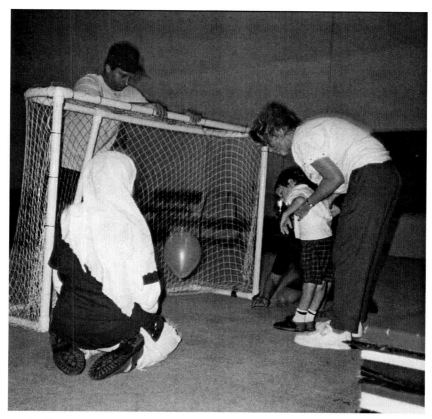

Figure 1.17. The interventionists facilitate a kicking activity with a young child with cerebral palsy.

or motor control. When teaching a child with a disability, DST can be applied by identifying a primary rate-limiter specific to the child's delay or disability (Sayers, Cowden, Newton, Warren, & Eason, 1996; Ulrich & Ulrich, 1993, 1995). For example, although infants with Down syndrome have a functional central nervous system, muscle hypotonicity is present. By increasing strength through individualized strength intervention, infants with Down syndrome were able to acquire independent upright locomotion (Sayers, et al., 1996) (see Figure 1.18). Lack of strength was the identified rate limiter that had prevented infants from walking independently.

To summarize the components of DST, development occurs during stability, instability, and phase shifts in the attractor states. This ensures that familiar movement patterns will emerge from specified

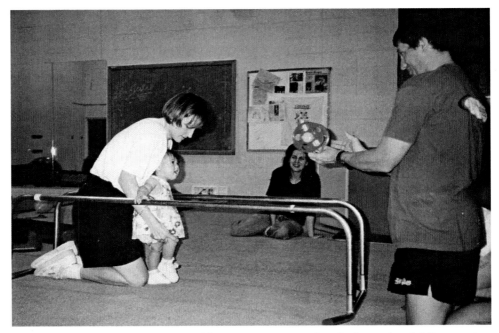

Figure 1.18. Flexion at the hips and knees is encouraged to facilitate the child's stepping movements, while verbal and visual motivation is provided. The child's Family Service Coordinator observes the intervention program.

conditions. Instability leads to a change as the child's system selects new methods of coordination. The new methods of stability are refined to increasing levels of efficiency. The contemporary views presented by Thelen provide support for early intervention and the designing of motor programs (Ulrich, Ulrich, Collier & Cole, 1995). Practice, repetition, and neurodevelopmental facilitation of movements impact a child's motor development. Multisensory stimulation as a component of early intervention programs influence avenues in the establishment of neural patterns, thus allowing for new behaviors to emerge from both internal and external collective interaction.

SUMMARY

This chapter provided a theoretical framework to distinguish traditional, neurodevelopmental, and contemporary theories. Professionals need a good understanding of the various theoretical perspectives which guide motor assessments and the development of intervention programs. Early theoretical principles developed throughout the 1900s should not be discounted as new philosophies emerge. Studies which encompass the motor development of infants and young children with delays cross over many disciplines including medical, developmental psychology, neuropsychology, early childhood, motor learning, motor development, physical education, special education, etc. (see Figure 1.19). Of paramount importance is that the movement professional establish a knowledge-base to direct assessment and intervention. Combinations of scientific attributes should be carefully selected. With the emergence of new theories, opportunities are presented to apply individualized research techniques to young children with delays or developmental disabilities. Ultimately, the clarity provided by the contemporary theories facilitates linking theory, assessment, and intervention (see Figure 1.20).

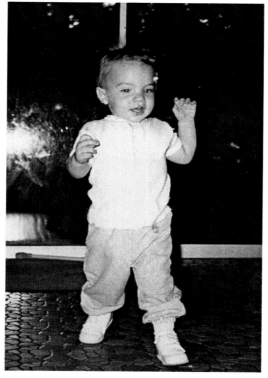

Figure 1.19. Through repeated cycles of action, a toddler maintains momentary upright position in attempting to take a few independent steps.

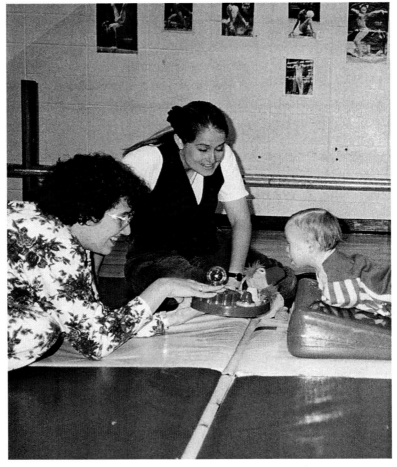

Figure 1.20. Multisensory information is available to the infant (re: Mom blows bubbles) as leg movement is facilitated.

REFERENCES

Ayres, A. J. (1972). *Sensory integration and learning disorders.* Los Angeles: Western Psychological Services.

Ayres, A. J. (1974). *The development of sensory integration theory and practice.* Dubuque, IA: Kendall/Hunt.

Ayres, A. J. (1980). *Sensory integration and the child.* Los Angeles: Western Psychological Services.

Ayres, A. J. (1989). *Sensory integration and praxis tests.* Los Angeles: Western Psychological Services.

Bayley, N. (1936). *The California infant scale of motor development.* Berkeley: University of California.

Bayley, N. (2006). *Bayley scales of infant and toddler development* (3rd ed.). San Antonio, TX: Harcourt.

Bernstein, N. A. (1967). *The coordination and regulation of movements.* New York: Pergamon Press.

Bobath, K., & Bobath, B. (1964). The facilitation of normal postural reactions and movements in the treatment of cerebral palsy. *Physiotherapy* (England), *50,* 246–262.

Cowden, J., & Torrey, C. (1995). A roadmap for assessing infants, toddlers, and preschoolers: The role of the adapted motor developmentalist. *Adapted Physical Activity Quarterly, 12* (1), 1–11.

Cratty, B. (1964). *Movement behavior and motor learning.* Philadelphia: Lea and Febiger.

Cratty, B. (1979). *Perceptual and motor development in infants and children.* Englewood Cliffs, NJ: Prentice Hall.

Crutchfield, C. A., & Barnes, M. R. (1993). *Motor control and motor learning in rehabilitation.* Atlanta, GA: Stokesville.

DeVries, R., & Kohlberg, L. (1990). *Constructivist early education: Overview and comparison with other programs.* Washington, DC: National Association for the Education of Young Children.

Dunn, J. M. & Leitschuh, C. A. (2006). *Special physical education* (8th ed.). Dubuque, IA: Kendall/Hunt.

Eichstaedt, C. B., & Kalakian, L. H. (1993). *Developmental/Adapted physical education.* New York: Macmillan.

Espenschade, A., & Eckert, H. (1980). *Motor development.* Columbus, OH: Merrill.

Fewell, R. R., & Glick, M. P. (1996). Program evaluation findings of an intensive early intervention program. *American Journal on Mental Retardation, 101* (3), 233–243.

Fiorentino, M. R. (1963). *Reflex testing methods for evaluating C.N.S. development.* Springfield, IL: Charles C Thomas.

Gallahue, D. L., & Ozmun, J. C. (2006). *Understanding motor development* (6th ed.). Boston: McGraw Hill.

Galloway, J. C., & Thelen, E. (2003). Feet first: Object exploration in young infants. *Infant behavior & Development, 27*(1), 107–113.

Gesell, A. (1928). *Infancy and human growth.* New York: Macmillan.

Gesell, A. (1939). Reciprocal interweaving in neuromotor development. *The Journal of Comparative Neurology, 70*(2), 161–180.

Gesell, A. (1945). *The embryology of behavior.* New York: Harper.

Gesell, A. (1946). The ontogenesis of infant behavior. In L. Carmichael (Ed.), *Manual of Child Psychology* (pp. 295–331). New York: Wiley.

Gesell, A. (1949). *Gesell developmental schedules.* New York: Psychological Corp.

Gesell, A. (1954). The ontogenesis of infant behavior. In L. Carmichael (Ed.). *Manual of Child Psychology* (2nd ed.) (pp. 335–373). New York: John Wiley & Son.

Gesell, A., & Ames, L. B. (1940). The ontogenetic organization of prone behavior in human infancy. *The Journal of Genetic Psychology, 56,* 247–263.

Gilfoyle, E., Grady, A., & Moore, J. (1981). *Children adapt.* Thorofare, NJ: Charles B. Slack.

Holle, B. (1981). *Motor development in children.* Oxford: Blackwell Scientific

Publications.

Kamm, K., Thelen, E., & Jensen, J. L. (1990). A dynamical systems approach to motor development. *Physical Therapy, 70,* 763–765.

Kelso, J. A. S. (Ed.) (1982). *Human motor behavior: An introduction.* Hillsdale, NJ.: Lawrence Erlbaum.

Knott, M., & Voss, D. E. (1968). *Proprioceptive neuromuscular facilitation: Patterns and techniques* (2nd ed.). New York: Harper and Row.

Lockman, J. J., & Thelen, E. (1993). Developmental biodynamics: Brain, body, behavior connections. *Child Development, 64,* 953–959.

Malina, R. (1975). *The first twenty years in man.* Minneapolis, MN: Burgess.

McGraw, M. B. (1932). From reflex to muscular control in the assumption of erect posture and ambulation in the human infant. *Child Development, 3,* 291–297.

McGraw, M. B. (1940). Neuromuscular development of the human infant as exemplified in the achievement of erect locomotion. *The Journal of Pediatrics, 17,* 747–771.

McGraw, M. B. (1945). *The neuromuscular maturation of the human infant.* New York: Columbia University Press.

McGraw, M. B. (1946). Maturation of behavior. In L. Carmichael (Ed.), *Manual of child psychology* (pp. 332–369). New York: Wiley.

Milani-Comparetti Motor Development Screening Test Manual (1987). Available from Meyers Children's Rehabilitation Institute, University of Nebraska Medical Center, 444 South 44th Street, Omaha, NE 68131-3795.

Milani-Comparetti, A., & Gidoni, E. (1967). Pattern analysis of motor development and its disorders. *Developmental Medicine and Child Neurology, 9,* 625–630.

Montessori, M. (1909/1964). *The Montessori method.* New York: Schocken Books.

Montessori, M. (1914/1965). *Dr. Montessori's own handbook.* New York: Schocken Books.

Montessori, M. (1936a/1956). *The child in the family.* New York: Avon Books.

Montessori, M. (1936b/1966). *The secret of childhood.* New York: Ballantine Books.

Montessori, M. (1949/1967). *The absorbent mind.* New York: Dell.

Moran, J. M., & Kalakian, L. H. (1974). *Movement experiences for the mentally retarded or emotionally disturbed child.* Minneapolis, MN: Burgess.

Parks, S. (2006). *Inside HELP.* Palo Alto, CA: VORT.

Payne, V., & Isaacs, I. D. (2005). *Human motor development: A lifespan approach.* (6th ed.). Blacklich, OH: McGraw Hill.

Piaget, J. (1951). *Play, dreams, and imitation in childhood.* New York: Norton.

Piaget, J. (1952). *The origins of intelligence in children.* New York: International Universities Press.

Piaget, J. (1985). *The equilibration of cognitive structures: The central problem of intellectual development.* Chicago: University of Chicago Press.

Rood, M. (1954). Neurophysiological reactions as a basis for physical therapy. *Physical Therapy Review, 34,* 444.

Rood, M. (1956). Neurophysiological mechanisms utilized in the treatment of neuromuscular dysfunction. *American Journal of Occupational Therapy, 10,* 220–224.

Sayers, L. K., Cowden, J. E., Newton, M., Warren, B., & Eason, B. (1996). Qualitative analysis of a pediatric strength intervention on the developmental stepping movements of infants with Down syndrome. *Adapted Physical Activity Quarterly, 13* (3), 247–268.

Seefelt, V. (1989). This is motor development. *Motor Development Academy Newsletter, 10,* 2–5.

Sherrill, C. (1981). *Adapted physical education and recreation: A multidisciplinary approach* (2nd. ed.) Dubuque, IA: Wm. C. Brown.

Sherrill, C. (1993). *Adapted physical activity, recreation, and sport: Crossdisciplinary and lifespan* (4th ed.). Dubuque, IA: Brown & Benchmark.

Sherrill, C. (1998). *Adapted physical activity, recreation, and sport: Crossdisciplinary and lifespan* (5th ed.). Madison, WI: WBC McGraw-Hill.

Sherrill, C. (2004). *Adapted physical activity, recreation, and sport: Crossdisciplinary and lifespan* (6th ed.). New York: McGraw-Hill.

Sherrington, C. S. (1906). *The integrative action of the nervous system.* New Haven: Yale University.

Shirley, M. M. (1931). *The first two years: A study of twenty-five babies,* Vol. I. Minneapolis: University of Minnesota Press.

Thelen, E. (1983). Learning to walk is still an "old" problem: A reply to Zelazo. *Journal of Motor Behavior, 15,* 139–161.

Thelen, E. (1985). Developmental origins of motor coordination: Leg movements in human infants. *Developmental Psychobiology, 18,* 1–22.

Thelen, E. (1987). The role of motor development in developmental psychology: A view of the past and an agenda for the future. In N. Eisenberg (Ed.), *Contemporary Topics in Developmental Psychology* (pp. 3–33). New York: John Wiley & Sons.

Thelen, E. (1989). Self-organization in developmental processes: Can systems approaches work? In M. Gunnar & E. Thelen (Eds.), *Systems and Development: The Minnesota Symposia in Child Psychology, 22,* (pp. 77–117). Hillsdale, NJ: Lawrence Erlbaum.

Thelen, E. (1992). Development as a dynamic system. *Current Directions in Psychological Science, 1*(6), 189–193.

Thelen, E. (1994). Three-month-old infants can learn task-specific patterns of inter-limb coordination. *Psychological Science, 5*(5), 280–285.

Thelen, E. (1995). Motor development: A new synthesis. *American Psychologist, 50*(2), 79–95.

Thelen, E., & Bates, E. (2003). Connectionism and dynamic systems: Are they really different? *Developmental Science, 6*(4), 378–391.

Thelen, E., & Cooke, D. W. (1987). The relation between newborn stepping and later locomotion: A new interpretation. *Developmental Medicine and Child Neurology, 29,* 380–393.

Thelen, E., & Fisher, D. M. (1982). Newborn stepping: An explanation for a "disappearing" reflex. *Developmental Psychology, 18,* 760–775.

Thelen, E., & Fisher, D. M. (1983a). From spontaneous to instrumental behavior: Kinematic analysis of movement changes during very early learning. *Child Development, 54,* 129–140.

Thelen, E., & Fisher, D. M. (1983b). The organization of spontaneous leg movements in newborn infants. *Journal of Motor Behavior, 15,* 353–377.

Thelen, E., Fisher, D. M., & Ridley-Johnson, R. (1984). The relationship between physical growth and a newborn reflex. *Infant Behavior and Development, 7,* 479–493.

Thelen, E., & Fogel, A. (1989). Toward an action-based theory of infant development. In J. Lockman & N. Hazen (Eds.), *Action in Social Context* (pp. 23–62). New York: Plenum.

Thelen, E., Kelso, J. A. S., & Fogel, A. (1987). Self-organizing systems and infant motor development. *Developmental Review, 7,* 39–65.

Thelen, E., & Smith, L. B. (1994). *A dynamic systems approach to the development of cognition and action.* Cambridge, MA: The MIT Press.

Thelen, E., & Ulrich B. D. (1991). Hidden skills: A dynamic systems analysis of treadmill stepping during the first year. *Monographs of the Society for Research in Child Development, 56,* (1, Serial no. 223).

Thelen, E., Ulrich, B. D., & Jensen, J. L. (1989). The developmental origins of locomotion. In M. H. Woollacott & A. Shumway-Cook (Eds.). *Development of posture and gait across the life span* (pp. 25–47). Columbia: University of South Carolina Press.

Ulrich, B. D., & Ulrich D. A. (1993). Dynamic systems approach to understanding motor delay in infants with Down syndrome. In G.J. P. Savelsbergh (Ed.), *The development of coordination in infancy* (pp. 445–457). North Holland: Elsevier Science Publishers.

Ulrich, B. D., & Ulrich D. A. (1995). Spontaneous leg movements of infants with Down syndrome and nondisabled infants. *Child Development, 66,* 1844–1855.

Ulrich, B. D., Ulrich, D. A., Collier, D. H., & Cole, E. L. (1995). Developmental shifts in the ability of infants with Down syndrome to produce treadmill steps. *Physical Therapy, 75* (1), 20–29.

Williams, H. (1983). *Perceptual and motor skills.* Englewood Cliffs, NJ: Prentice-Hall.

Chapter 2

ORGANIZATION OF THE NERVOUS SYSTEM

Chapter Objectives: After studying this chapter, the reader will be able to:
1. Give the purpose of the central nervous system;
2. Diagram and explain the simple reflex arc;
3. Define the principle of segmental innervation;
4. List and give the function of the major parts of the central nervous system;
5. Diagram and explain the perceptual motor response theory model and explain each component and its effect on movement;
6. Discuss the importance of each of the sensory systems in relation to motor output.

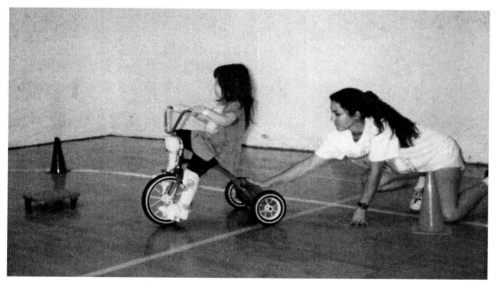

Figure 2.1. Interactions of all subsystems with the CNS are demonstrated by a young child with spina bifida pedaling a tricycle through an obstacle course.

This chapter presents a discussion of the basic organization and neuroanatomy of the nervous system and the Perceptual Motor Response Model. The nervous system is very complex. The intention is to provide a brief overview highlighting the parts of the central nervous system (CNS) which most affect motor control.

DEVELOPMENT OF THE NERVOUS SYSTEM

The nervous system receives and responds to all stimuli. Its primary purpose is to govern and coordinate all activities of the body. The CNS governs movement and sensation while the autonomic nervous system controls vital functions like the heart and blood pressure, bladder and bowel control, sexual activity, and temperature.

Damage to the nervous system may be caused by genetic factors, malnutrition and poor prenatal health care of the mother, increased levels of alcohol and drug levels of the mother, insufficient oxygen during the birth process, and trauma during the delivery process causing intraventricular hemorrhage. Primary signs of congenital nervous system involvement include mental retardation, abnormal muscle tone (e.g., hypertonicity or hypotonicity), delayed sensorimotor responses, and paralysis of one or more extremities. Of all the congenital defects, over 50 percent will involve the nervous system. This estimate has probably increased in recent years since Fetal Alcohol Syndrome (FAS) has become a leading cause of mental retardation and FAS affects brain growth (K. Hymbaugh, Center for Disease Control, Atlanta, GA. Personal Communication, December 13, 1996. Available E-mail: kxh5@CEHBDDD.EM.CDC.GOV).

The nervous system is approximately 85 percent complete at birth and continues to develop throughout early childhood. Major motor milestones cannot be accomplished until the process of myelination is completed. For example, myelination of the pyramidal tract occurs at 12 months, the time when the motor patterns of standing alone and walking should mature.

Motor maturation is dependent on the development of myelin, the innermost fatty covering of nerve fibers. Myelin formation is vital because it increases the velocity of nerve conduction and adds efficiency to the nervous system. Myelin is not essential in all cases for nerve conduction; however, it is required to some degree for the development of delicate and precise movements. In comparison to the rest of the nervous system, myelin formation begins late at approximately 12 weeks gestation. Myelination begins with the cervical spinal cord. The major motor pathways for voluntary movements, pyramidal and extrapyramidal tracts, do not begin myelination until just before birth and continue into the second year of life. The sensory systems that mature earliest (around 17 weeks gestation) are touch and deep pressure, vestibular, and kinesthetic (Burt, 1993; House & Pansky, 1967).

Neural tissue has the fastest growth rate of all systems of the body. Therefore, the nervous system of the newborn is functioning adequately at birth. The newborn responds to light intensity, moves and turns the head to seek sufficient oxygen, shows protective reactions to pain, and searches for the mother's nipple to receive nourishment.

The functional unit of the nervous system is the nerve cell or **neuron**. Neurons are capable of receiving and sending information. A neuron is composed of the cell body with numerous extensions of the cell specialized for reception of information (**dendrites**) and a single long process (**axon**) for the transmission of a nerve impulse (**action potential**). Communication between neurons takes place at a synapse through the exchange of a chemical message or neurotransmitter. **Sensory** (**afferent**) neurons relay information from the end receptors (skin, muscles, tendons, joints, organs) to the spinal cord and brain (CNS). **Motor** (**efferent**) neurons convey messages from the CNS to the muscles resulting a reflex, reaction, or motor skill (Burt, 1993; House & Pansky, 1967; Noback, 2005).

The completion of a neural circuit is termed reflex arc. The **reflex arc** is composed of a receptor, afferent input neuron, connecting neurons (intercalated or internuncial neurons), or internuncial neuron, an efferent output neuron, and a muscle or organ that produces activity. A simple reflex may involve only two neurons and one joint. A more complex reflex arc involves numerous neurons resulting in movements of the whole body. The earliest reflex responses may be elicited from the embryo at approximately 8 weeks gestation. Figure 2.2 provides a diagram of the simple reflex arc (Brown, 1980; Gonzales, Myers, Downey, & Darling, 2001; Kolb & Whishaw, 2003).

Spinal Cord

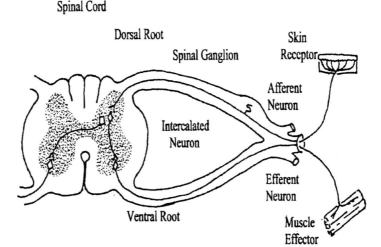

Figure 2.2. Simple reflex arc (Adapted from Brown, D., 1980. *Neurosciences for allied health therapies.* St. Louis: Mosby.

SPINAL CORD DEVELOPMENT AND FUNCTIONS

Reflex activity usually involves more than one segment of the spinal cord. There are 31 pairs of **spinal nerves** (eight cervical, twelve thoracic, five lumbar, five sacral, and one coccygeal). Each spinal nerve receives sensory information from a particular area of the skin and the underlying muscles. Each spinal nerve is composed of **dorsal roots** (sensory nerve fibers) and **ventral roots** (motor nerve fibers). The concept of **"segmental innervation"** (see Figure 2.3) involves an area of the skin supplied by dendrites from one dorsal root ganglia projecting into one spinal cord segment and one ventral root of the spinal cord and the underlying muscles or portions of muscle. Stimulation of the surface of skin tissue may be used to help activate this muscle tissue. Figure 2.3 provides a diagram displaying process of segmental innervation (Brown, 1980; Kolb & Whishaw, 2003). Figure 2.4 provides a pictorial diagram of the distribution of spinal nerves.

An understanding of the nature of spinal paralysis caused by injury, disease, or congenital birth defect is presented in relation to individual assessment and program intervention. The severity of loss of muscular functions depends on the level of spinal cord lesion. The higher the lesion occurs on the spinal cord, the greater the loss of muscular and other bodily functions. Paralysis may be complete or incomplete.

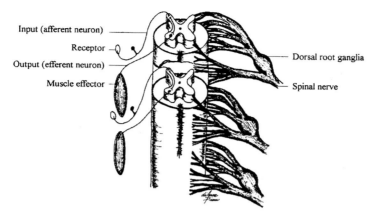

Figure 2.3. Segmental innervation. (Adapted from Brown, D., 1980. *Neurosciences for allied health therapies.* St. Louis: Mosby.)

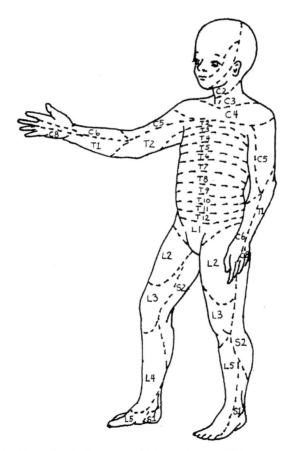

Figure 2.4. Distribution of spinal nerves. (Adapted from Noback, C., 2005. *The human nervous system: Structure and function.* Totowa, NJ: Humana Press.)

Partial or incomplete spinal cord damage may result in muscular weakening conditions. Figure 2.5 provides a pictorial design of the 31 pair of spinal nerves and indicates examples of functions which may occur at each level. Assessment of the strengths and weaknesses of individuals to prepare an individualized intervention program will assist the child in achieving the highest level of functional mobility (see Figures 7.2 and 7.3). In addition, alternatives for walking should be taught so that the child may later select methods of locomotion based on choice and challenge of physical activities.

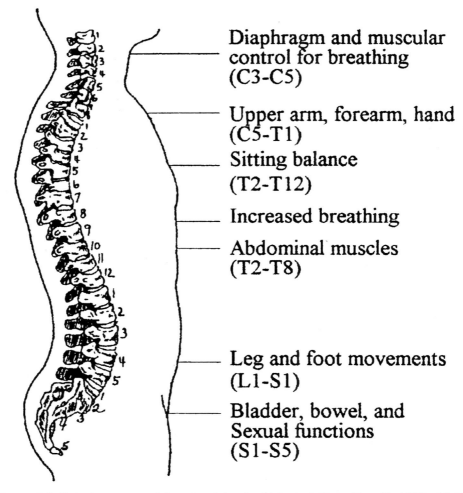

Diaphragm and muscular control for breathing (C3-C5)

Upper arm, forearm, hand (C5-T1)

Sitting balance (T2-T12)

Increased breathing

Abdominal muscles (T2-T8)

Leg and foot movements (L1-S1)

Bladder, bowel, and Sexual functions (S1-S5)

Figure 2.5. Spinal nerves and functional levels. (Adapted. from Sherrill, 1993. *Adapted physical activity, recreation, and sport: Crossdisciplinary and lifespan.* (4th ed.). Dubuque, IA: Brown & Benchmark.)

CRANIAL NERVES

A brief synopsis of the **cranial nerves** is included since trauma at birth is stressful to the newborn and neurological examinations entail assessment of the functional components (Burt, 1993; Ensher & Clark, 1994; Fenichel, 2005; House & Pansky, 1967). The birthing process can be a major trauma for the neonate. The cranial nerves are exposed to strong constriction pressures and temporary loss of function of the nerves may occur. However, functions are usually reestablished within a few weeks.

Cranial nerves considered as special senses include the olfactory (I), optic (II), and vestibulocochlear (VIII). **The olfactory (I)** nerve provides the sense of smell. Trauma to the head can cause loss of this special sense. Temporary loss of smell involving infection of the nasal passages due to sinusitis may be a problem in young children, especially congestion associated with Down syndrome. The second cranial nerve is the **optic nerve II** and the primary nerve for the visual modality. The optic nerve connects directly to the retina, therefore full-term newborns respond to light intensity, the color red, and facial features.

Cranial nerves III (oculomotor), IV (trochlear) and VI (abducens) have functions involving the muscular movements of the eye. **Oculomotor (III)** governs all of the extrinsic ocular muscles except the lateral rectus and superior oblique. Symptoms of disease or damage to this nerve are noticeable by the eye looking downward and outward with no convergence. This nerve also governs the pupil of the eye and its constriction in response to light. The **trochlear (IV)** cranial nerve innervates the superior oblique muscles and symptoms of dysfunction involve the eye tending to look slightly upward. The abducens (VI) nerve governs the lateral rectus muscle which turns the eye inward.

The **trigeminal (V)** nerve governs pain, temperature, and touch innervation of the face and the anterior two-thirds of the tongue affecting the chewing process. Trauma during birth occurring to the fifth and sixth cranial nerves can cause Erb's palsy, paralysis of shoulder and upper arm muscles and Klumpke's paralysis of the lower arm. **Cranial nerve VII (facial)** provides innervation to the muscles for facial expression. Paralysis of facial muscles is Bell's palsy. **Acoustic nerve VIII** is associated with loss of hearing and deafness. Most full term newborns respond to intensity and pitch of sound. **Cranial** nerve IX (**glossopharyngeal**) along with V (trigeminal) are responsible for swallowing, sucking, palate, and tongue functions. The **vagus nerve (X)** governs circulation, heart rate, blood pressure, and smooth muscle tissue of the trachea, bronchi, and esophagus. **Cranial nerve XI (accessory)** innervates some areas related to swallowing and muscles of the neck requiring flexion and turning of the head, primarily the sternocleidomastoid and trapezius muscles. **The hypoglossal (XII)** is responsible for all muscles of the tongue. Table 2.1 provides condensed definitions of the cranial nerve functions.

Table 2.1. Cranial Nerves.

Nerve	*Function*
Olfactory I	Sense of smell
Optic II	Primary nerve for visual modality
Oculomotor III	Extrinsic muscular movements of the eyes with the exception of the lateral rectus and superior oblique
Trochlear IV	Muscular movements of the superior oblique
Trigeminal V	Governs sensations of pain, temperature and touch; innervation of face and tongue affecting chewing
Abducens VI	Lateral rectus muscular movements of the eye
Facial VII	Facial expressions (e.g., smile, frown)
Acoustic VIII	Sense of hearing
Glossopharyngeal IX	Swallowing, sucking, and movements of tongue and palate
Vagus X	Governs circulation, heart rate, blood pressure, and smooth muscle tissue of the trachea, bronchi, and esophagus
Accessory XI	Flexor muscles of the neck, turning of head, assists with with swallowing
Hypoglossal XII	All muscles of the tongue

CENTRAL NERVOUS SYSTEM

The nervous system is composed of the **CNS** (brain and spinal cord) and the **peripheral nervous system** (31 pair of spinal nerves, 12 pair of cranial nerves), and the autonomic nervous system. From the least to the most complex, the major centers of the CNS are the spinal cord, medulla, pons, brain stem, midbrain, reticular activating system, cerebellum, thalamus, hypothalamus, basal ganglia, and the cerebrum or cerebral cortex. The **corpus callosum** connects the right and left cerebral hemispheres. Figure 2.6 provides a view of the midsagittal section of the brainstem, cerebellum, and cerebrum.

The **brain stem** is an upward extension of the spinal cord subdivided into the medulla, pons, and midbrain (however, the midbrain

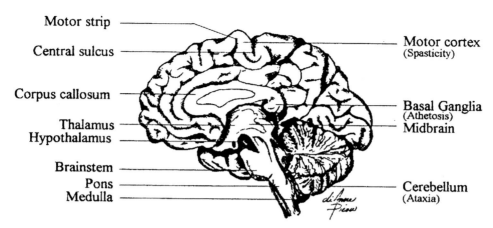

Figure 2.6. Midsagittal section of brainstem, cerebellum, and cerebrum. (Adapted from Truex, R. & Carpenter, M., 1969. *Human neuroanatomy* (6th ed.). Baltimore, MD: Williams & Wilkins.)

may be discussed separately by many authors). Ascending and descending nerve pathways pass through the brain stem affecting the degree of individual alertness. Both facilitory and suppressor areas are located in the brain stem. The brain stem governs reflex activity and integrates muscle tone. The control centers for the sense modalities are located in the brain stem with the exception of vision and smell. The **reticular activating system (RAS)** is formulated in this area and is comprised of the medulla, pons, and midbrain. The RAS serves to screen incoming sensory stimulation inhibiting some sensory input and processing other information. Alertness, attention, arousal, reciprocal innervation, and wakefulness are selective functions of the RAS.

The **medulla oblongata** is basically an upper extension of the spinal cord as it enters the brain. Anatomically, it is only about one inch long and the approximate diameter of a pencil. Ascending and descending sensory and motor tracts pass through the medulla; thus it serves as a synaptic relay station for all data. The nuclei for cranial nerves VIII, IX, X, XI, and XII are located in the medulla.

The **pons** is located above the medulla and forms a "bridge of fibers" connecting the medulla to the cerebellum. The nuclei of cranial nerves V through VIII are located in the pons. The **fourth ventricle** forms a cavity located between the pons, medulla, and cerebellum allowing for cerebrospinal fluid to circulate in the appropriate manner. The functions of the pons are important to head, neck and eye control,

control of equilibrium, and the regulation of coordination associated with attaining upright posture. Major spinal tracts associated with the pons and medulla are the spinocerebellar and the vestibulocochlear tracts.

The **midbrain** is the portion of the brain between the pons and the cerebral hemispheres composed of the superior and inferior **colliculi**. The superior and inferior colliculi are involved with visual and auditory reflexes respectively. The **cerebral aqueduct** connects the third and fourth ventricles located in the midbrain and can become obstructed easily. The primary function of the midbrain is to serve as a transmitting station for stimulation of the righting and postural reactions. If there is trauma to brain tissue, intraventricular hemorrhage may occur causing the ventricular cavities to fill with fluids which interfere with the ventricular systems primary function of circulation of the cerebrospinal fluid.

The **cerebellum** is the second largest portion of the brain. It is located posterior to the medulla and pons. It is believed that the cerebellum receives stimuli from all of the sensory modalities. Its primary function is to regulate muscular coordination for balance and integrate postural and equilibrium reactions. Both ascending and descending spinal tracts pass through the cerebellum controlling fast vs. slow movements, jerky vs. smooth coordination and the precise starting and stopping of movements. The cerebellum is sometimes referred to as the "little brain" because it provides for the automatic phase of movements that no longer require conscious thought.

The **thalamus** and **hypothalamus** serve as relay stations for all sensory impulses going to the cerebrum with the exception of the sense of smell. More specifically, the thalamus organizes and integrates sensory impulses and responds to the emotions of fear, rage, and pleasant or unpleasant sensations. The hypothalamus has a variety of functions including the following: (a) regulation of emotions and integration of autonomic nervous system responses, (b) temperature control, (c) water balance, (d) food intake and gastric secretions, (e) heart rate, and (f) expression of emotions.

The **basal ganglia** is a group of nuclei (e.g., caudate nucleus, globus pallidus, putamen) that regulate and modulate cortical information from almost every area of the cerebral hemispheres. Neural circuits from the cerebrum are directly involved in information processing of motor activity. The primary motor, premotor, and somatosensory areas of the "motorstrip" and the posterior parietal motor area are involved in preparation, planning, and execution of motor activity. This complex is at the base of the brain or located just below the cortex. Children with basal ganglia damage or lesions, as with cerebellar damage, are not paralyzed but have difficulty with the coordination of movements. A variety of disorders is associated with basal ganglia pathology and is classified into two categories with opposite symptomatology. **Akinesia** (lack of movement) and **hypertonia** (muscle rigidity) formulate one category and **dyskinesia** (abnormal movement) and **hypotonia** (muscle flaccidity) compose the second category. Disorders associated with the basal ganglia include Parkinson's disease, athetoid cerebral palsy, and Huntington's chorea.

The **cerebrum** or **cerebral cortex** is the largest portion of the human brain and is divided into two halves (hemispheres). It is the main center for voluntary movement, learning, perception, memory, and communication. The cerebrum can be divided into three areas: (a) afferent (sensory) areas, (b) integrative (association) areas, and (c) efferent (motor) areas. The pyramidal and extrapyramidal systems are the major pathways for movement control. The **pyramidal system** originates from pyramid-shaped cells of Betz of the cortex in Brodmann's area 4 which is anterior to the central sulcus. The pyramidal tract once was referred to as the corticospinal tract but current research (Burt, 1993; Shumway-Cook & Woollacott, 2001) indicated that additional nerve fibers (e.g., corticobulbar tract, corticoreticular tract) compose the system. The extrapyramidal system, which also originates in the motor strip of the cerebrum, travels in close association with the pyramidal tract. The **extrapyramidal system** includes the vestibulospinal, rubrospinal, and reticulospinal tracts. Although the pyramidal and extrapyramidal systems do not work independently of each other the pyramidal system stimulates or initiates muscular activity and is more responsible for precise movements necessary for fine and skillful coordination. The extrapyramidal system is more related to movements of automatic control and postural reactions. Pathological damage to the pyramidal system causes **spasticity**, a problem of overexcitibility or hypertonicity. Damage to the extrapyramidal system causes **athetosis** which is characterized by excessive movements. **Ataxia**, characterized by general incoordination, may be an upper motor neuron problem or a pathological disorder of the cerebellum (Burt, 1993; Downey & Darling, 1971; House & Pansky, 1967; Kolb &

Whishaw, 2003; Noback, 2005).

Brodmann's Cytoarchitectural Map (Peele, 1961) of the human cortex is used to define specific areas as related to function. Brodmann's area 4 (motor strip), areas 6 and 8 (premotor areas), areas 3, 1, and 2 (primary somatosensory), and area 17 (primary visual) are denoted in Figure 2.7. Area 4 located in the frontal lobe of the brain is related to fine and gross motor control. The pyramidal and extrapyramidal pathways originate in the area of the "motor strip" of the cerebral hemisphere. If pathological damage occurs in area 4, the result will be a condition termed **apraxia**, the inability to initiate purposive movements. Sensory motor receptors are functioning appropriately; however, associative neural pathways or cortical areas are unable to correctly interpret the sensory signals. Dysfunction within this area may also cause spasticity or grand mal (generalized tonic-clonic) seizures. The premotor areas (6, 8) also control purposive movements and the development of motor skills. Lesions in these areas cause problems with the coordination of movements of the eyes and head. In addition, other changes that may occur include alterations in memory, thinking, abstract reasoning, and unpredictable emotional and personality behaviors. Pathological damage to Broca's area 44 may cause motor or **speech apraxia**.

The primary somatosensory areas (3, 1, 2) are responsible for the interpretation of most skin sensations. In addition, two conditions which may result from damage in these areas include **agnosia** and **astereognosis**. **Agnosia**, the process of knowing, is a result of the failure to recognize familiar objects or past experiences. **Astereognosis** is a condition in which sensory input of the tactile vestibular-kinesthetic modalities results in the child not being able to identify familiar objects through feel and manipulation.

Brodmann's areas 41 and 42 receive auditory stimuli from the inner ear and areas 17 and 18 receive impulses from the optic nerve pathways for processing of visual information. **Aphasia** is a pathological condition which can be sensory, motor, or both and results in the child having difficulty understanding written or spoken words. **Aphasias** relate to the processing of cerebral cortex information and sensory input stimuli. Learning disorders or delays are often referred to as **dyslexia** (reading difficulties) or **dysgraphia** (writing disorders) (Auxter, Pyfer, & Huettig, 2005; Sherrill, 1993).

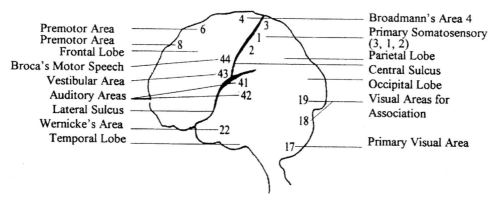

Figure 2.7. Brodman's cytoarchitectural map–Lateral view. (Adapted from Peele, T. L., 1961. *The neuroanatomical basis for clinical neurology.* New York: McGraw-Hill.)

PERCEPTUAL MOTOR RESPONSE THEORY MODEL

An understanding of how an individual receives and interprets a message and initiates movement is explained through the Perceptual Motor Response Theory Model (Figure 2.8). The sensory systems provide input to the CNS. Each system will be discussed in detail relating the importance of multisensory stimulation of infants and young children.

Sensory Systems and Sensory Input

Sensation is the reception of internal and external stimuli for which the primary purpose is to provide information about the functioning of the body. There are 10 sensory systems that provide sensory (afferent) input to the CNS. The sense modalities that will be discussed are touch and pressure (tactile), vestibular, auditory, visual, and kinesthetic.

Each sensory system has its own end receptors that must receive stimulation and specific pathways that transmit information throughout the CNS. System receptors respond to different sensory stimuli with specificity of intensity (Burt, 1993; Cech & Martin, 2002; Seaman & DePauw, 1995; Sherrill, 1993). The two oldest systems are the tactile and vestibular, which provide the most basic forms of physical and emotional security. The sense modalities develop in utero in the following sequence: tactile, vestibular, smell, auditory, vision, taste, and kinesthetic (Cech & Martin, 2002).

PERCEPTUAL MOTOR RESPONSE THEORY MODEL

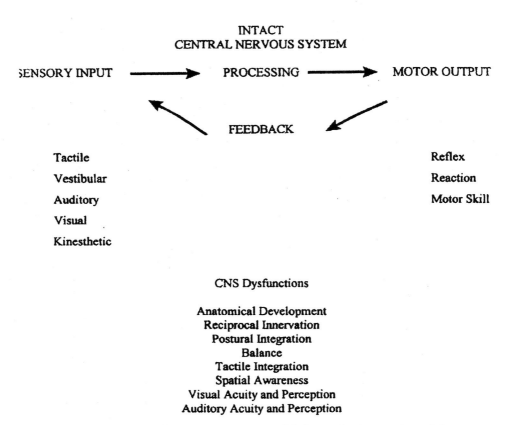

Figure 2.8. The perceptual motor response model shows the interaction of the sensory systems with central nervous system processing and the resulting motor output.

Tactile Modality

The tactile system, the first to develop, is functioning by 17 weeks gestation. It is probably the most developed sensory system at birth (Cech & Martin, 2002; Widerstrom, Mowder, & Sandall, 1991). In the newborn, touch provides the infant with a means of interacting with his environment and is the "primary system for making contact with the external world" (Fisher, Murray & Bundy, 1991, p. 108).

The skin serves as the organ for many different receptors for touch, deep pressure massage, temperature, and pain. The tactile modality has six special sensory receptors which are as follows: (a) **free nerve**

endings located in the skin, joint capsules, tendons, and ligaments responding to pain and temperature; (b) **hair follicles** located in deep temperature; dermal layers responding to hair arrangement and pain; (c) **Meissner's corpuscles** located in the papillae of skin responding to light touch; (d) **Pacinian corpuscles** located in the subcutaneous tissue responding to deep pressure and vibration; (e) **Krause's end bulb** located in the skin responding to temperature; (f) **Merkel's disc** located in hair follicles and sensitive to low intensity as well as velocity of touch; and (g) **Ruffini ending** located in the joint capsules and connective tissue responding to deep massage (Cech & Martin, 2002; Coren, Ward, & Enns, 2004; Fisher et al., 1991; Reisman, 1987; Royeen & Lane, 1991).

Discussions of the tactile sensory modality often involve association with proprioceptive sensation. Ayres (1989) referred to the combination of input from both modalities as **somatosensory processing**. The interaction of these two modalities is extremely important to the infant's early learning and subsequent development. The tactile modality provides the infant with the first avenues for communication or nonverbal language. A premature or high-risk infant's initial experiences with touch and interaction with the new world may involve encounters associated with pain and discomfort. An infant who must be hospitalized in a Neonatal Intensive Care Unit (NICU) is bombarded with negative and excessive exposure to touch and overstimulation by medical caregivers, high-pitched auditory stimuli, and painful treatment procedures (Ensher & Clark, 1994; Rossetti, 1986; Widerstrom et al., 1991).

A result of these first negative sensations may cause the infant to exhibit difficulties associated with **tactile integration** and cause later problems of tactile defensiveness and poor tactile discrimination. **Tactile defensiveness** is defined as a negative response to certain tactile stimuli. Infants and young children may avoid certain textures, pull away from anticipated interactions involving touch, or avoid play activities involving contact with another child. **Tactile discrimination** is the ability to recognize, perceive and organize information involving touch, for example, soft or hard, wet or dry, food discrimination, and body localization. Poor tactile discrimination contributes to poor body orientation or schema and poor form and symbol discrimination (Ayres, 1989; Cech & Martin, 2002; Fisher et al., 1991). The sensitivity of the tactile modality should be recognized through assessment and

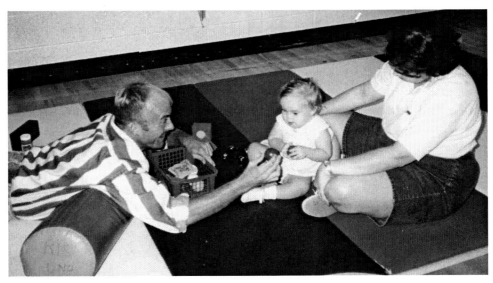

Figure 2.9. This young child uses the tactile and visual modalities during fine motor manipulation of objects held in midline.

activities should be carefully planned for meeting the individual needs of each child (see Figure 2.9).

Vestibular Modality

The vestibular modality is the sensory system which is responsible for the development of equilibrium and balance. The vestibular system is traditionally viewed as having three major functions: (a) awareness of body position and movement in space; (b) postural tone and equilibrium; and (c) stabilization of the eyes in space during head movements (Fisher et al., 1991). The sensory receptors for the vestibular system are found in the inner ear and are the semicircular canals, the utricle, and the saccule. The organs pertaining to static equilibrium include the vestibule, utricle, and saccule and the receptors for dynamic balance include the three semicircular canals in the inner ear. The receptors are stimulated by movement of the head, change of the head in relation to space, and the normal pull of gravity (see Figure 2.10). The vestibular system is intimately connected with the proprioceptive system, the primary method of receiving sensory information (Auxter et al., 2005; Eichstaedt & Kalakian, 1993; Gallahue & Ozmun, 2006; Payne & Isaacs, 2005; Sherrill, 1993).

The infant must first gain control over the musculature of the head and neck in order to gain stability. The development of balance in young children includes the maturation of the equilibrium and righting reactions. **Righting** means to bring the head and body into alignment with each other and in respect to other body segments and the surrounding environment. The Progression of Balance Development in Chapter 6 details the development and assessment of balance in infants and young children.

Problems associated with balance are most often noticed when a child appears clumsy or awkward among his typical peers. A. Jean Ayres (1972) first introduced the concept of vestibular system dysfunctions and the process of sensory integration in her classic text, *Sensory Integration and Learning Disorders.* According to Fisher et al. (1991), "Vestibular processing disorders have been associated with learning disabilities and motor coordination deficits and treatment directed toward the vestibular system has been advocated as basis for remediating the underlying problem" (p. 72).

Infants with immature or delayed development will also exhibit problems associated with vestibular system processing. Delayed inhibition of primitive reflexes, normalization of muscle tone, poor equilibrium and righting reactions, and difficulties with visual tracking are

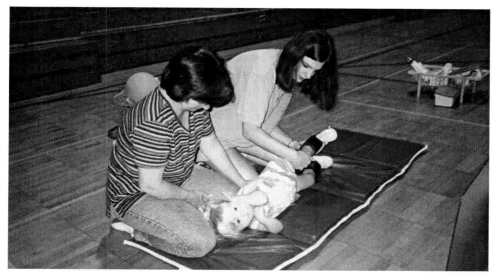

Figure 2.10. The vestibular system of this young child is stimulated as her mother and the movement specialist assists her with rolling.

clinical assessment signs indicating possible problems with sensory integration and vestibular processing. These problems will interfere with the development of later mobility skills associated with the acquisition of mature static and dynamic balance (see Figure 2.11). In addition, tactile defensiveness and weaknesses in tactile discrimination, visual motor coordination, and form and space perception indicate problems in vestibular-proprioceptive processing.

Auditory Modality

The auditory sensory system follows in development after the tactile and vestibular systems at approximately 25–33 weeks gestation. During the fetal period the auditory system is stimulated by external sounds such as the mother's speech and heartbeat. The sensory receptors are the inner ear cochlea and the Organ of Corti. Energy is transmitted through the eighth cranial nerve into the temporal lobe of the brain. Full-term infants have the capacity to discriminate a wide range of frequencies and intensities of sound (see Figure 2.12).

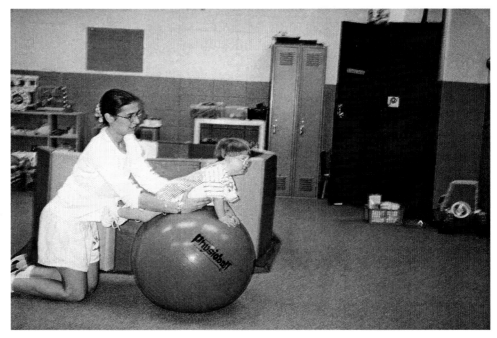

Figure 2.11. This vestibular activity stimulates head righting and protective extension.

The risk of hearing impairment increases according to the degree of prematurity, low birth weight, and other associated conditions such as intracranial hemorrhage, maternal rubella during pregnancy, cytomegalovirus infection, and hyperbilirubinemia. Brodmann's area 41 and 42 receive nerve impulses from the receptors of the inner ear. Auditory perceptual difficulties such as auditory reception, sequential memory, figure-background phenomenon and discrimination may also increase in risk with the degree of developmental delay.

Visual Modality

By the end of the 24th week gestation, the anatomy of the eye is almost complete and is presumably capable of functioning. The ocular muscles that control eye movements are not fully developed at birth. Often the newborn exhibits random movements of each eye or **strabismus** (crossed-eyes), an attribute which should greatly diminish or disappear during the first week of development. **Visual acuity** is difficult to determine at birth. The visual modality develops slowly throughout the first year of life. During the first week after birth the full-term infant is capable of processing complex visual information

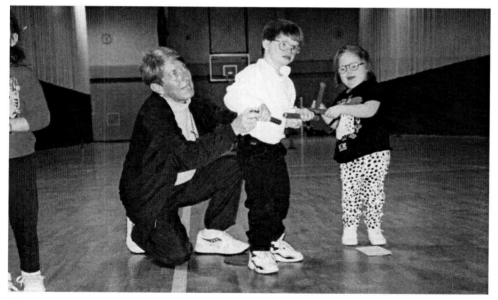

Figure 2.12. Rhythmic lummi stick tapping to music enhances auditory development and eye-hand coordination.

and responding to the human face, brightly colored objects, and high degrees of contrast in light. The visual system is best evaluated during the neonate period by observing tracking skills, visual attentiveness, fixation, and visual preference (Ensher & Clark, 1994; Haith, 1966; Payne & Isaacs, 2005; Widerstrom, et al., 1991).

Any discussion of vision should include the importance of the anatomy of the eye. The eye is basically an extension of the forebrain and is an inseparable part of the CNS. Three of the twelve pair of cranial nerves is necessary for muscular actions of visual motor processes. The sensory receptors for the visual modality include two **photoreceptors**, the **rods**, which provide input for black and white vision (twilight vision) and the **cones**, which provide color vision and acuity.

Getman (1952) proposed that 85 to 90 percent. of a child's learning is acquired through visual processes. Sherrill (1986)   supported this claim, "After school age is reached, approximately 90 percent of what the normally functioning child learns comes from visual input" (p. 98). This statement supports the critical importance of utilizing a multisensory approach to curricula intervention (see Figures 2.13 and 2.14). Young children who experienced delayed development at birth, even

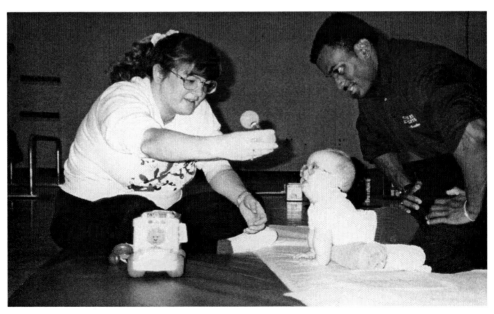

Figure 2.13. Visual and auditory stimulation are provided by the Mom to her child as the movement specialist provides further intervention suggestions.

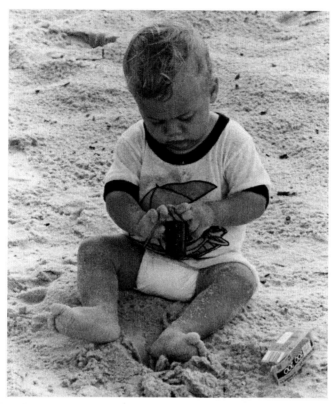

Figure 2.14. Eye-hand coordination is needed as this young child tries to remove and replace the lid of a small container.

those with normal IQ, are at risk for later learning disabilities especially in the area of visual integration and motor function.

Premature and low birth weight infants are often hospitalized in NICU and require ventilator oxygen therapy. The oxygen therapy may cause **retinopathy of prematurity (ROP)**. Respiratory distress and mechanical ventilation appear to be related to poor performance in visual perception including visual motor recognition, memory, attention, pattern recognition, discrimination, figure-ground differentiation and cross modality transfer (Morante, Dubowitz, Levene, & Dubowitz, 1982; Thompson, Fagan, & Fulker, 1991). Dubowitz, Dubowitz, and Morante (1980) also found visual fixation or tracking and acuity problems in premature infants with intraventricular hemorrhage. It is probable that a high percentage of young children who were delayed at birth will experience some type of visual perception and prehension problems causing later learning disabilities (DeGangi & Greenspan, 1988; Pederson, Evans, Chance, Bento, & Fox, 1988; Saigal, Szatmari, Rosenbaum, Campbell, & King, 1991).

Kinesthetic Modality

The kinesthetic modality is often referred to as **proprioception** and is defined as the awareness of active movement of one's own body in space. The sensory receptors for this modality are located in the skin and deeper tissue, the muscles, tendons, and joints, and hair cells located in the semicircular canals, utricle, saccule, and cochlea of the inner ear.

Kinesthetic perception is often combined with tactile and vestibular input (see Figure 2.15). Labyrinthine and proprioceptive signals con-

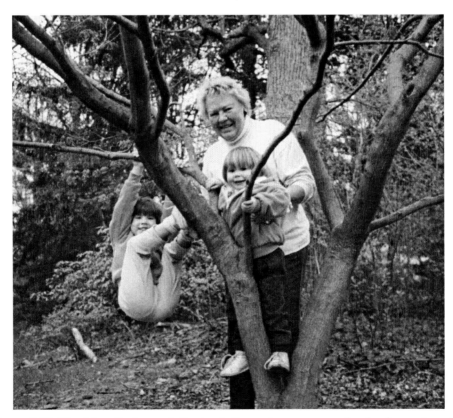

Figure 2.15. The kinesthetic modality is challenged as one preschooler hangs inverted and another balances with assistance.

verge to provide messages related to conscious awareness of body orientation. Ayres (1978) found that children with sensory integrative disorders often exhibit problems with bilateral coordination, equilibrium and balance, and planned motor sequences. Young children with delayed development may benefit from coactive, guided, and repetitive movement patterns which allow them to develop an "internal awareness or feel" for the motor skill (see Figure 2.16).

INTACT CENTRAL NERVOUS SYSTEM

The Perceptual Motor Theory Model assumes that the individual has an intact CNS. If the individual has delayed or abnormal motor development, the motor output responses of a reflex, reaction, or skill may be inappropriate, delayed, or absent. Several disorders of the CNS have been defined throughout the previous discussion of the sensory motor modalities. Refer to Chapter 4 for discussion of other syndromes or dysfunctions.

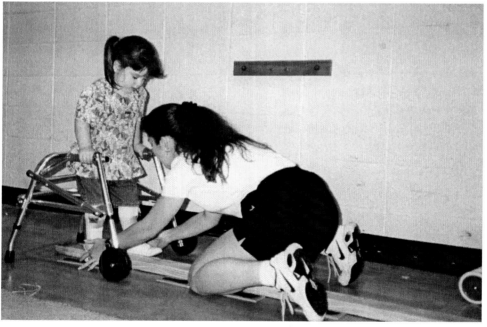

Figure 2.16. The interventionist provides coactive movement to assist a young child with stepping movement.

MOTOR OUTPUT

Motor Output as a Reflex

The reflex action is present at birth and is thought to be a prepro-grammed automatic mechanism for movement (Hanson, 1996). In the neonate the primary or primitive reflexes appear to provide prepara-tion for later progressive development such as rolling, sitting, crawling, creeping, standing, and walking. Typical neurodevelopmental reflex-ive maturation of the CNS progresses from spinal cord level, to brain stem, midbrain, and cortical levels. Fiorentino (1963) stressed that "early referral of patients for reflex therapy cannot be over-empha-sized" (p. 4).

In typical development, **primitive reflexes** should be present at birth resulting in predominate flexor and extensor movements (see Figure 2.17). These spinal cord and brain stem reflexes should dimin-ish or be inhibited by the CNS so higher righting or equilibrium reac-

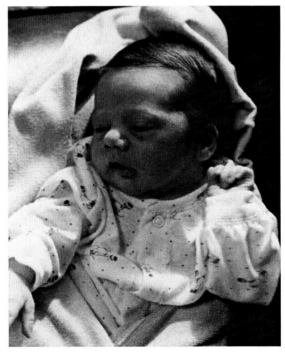

Figure 2.17. The asymmetrical tonic neck reflex (ATNR) occurred as this 6-week-old infant turned his head to the side.

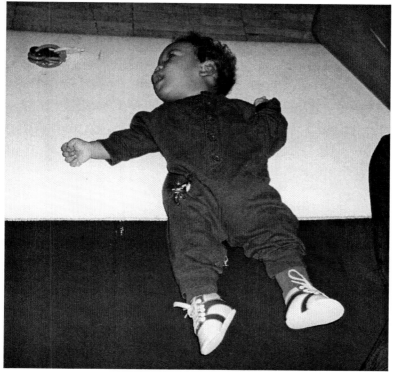

Figure 2.18. Residual ATNR prevents this young child from rolling over to his toy.

tions may be clearly revealed. When there is CNS dysfunction causing abnormal development, the primitive reflexes will be retained and will interfere with the appearance of the equilibrium reactions and the motor development patterns of rolling, sitting, crawling, creeping, standing, and walking (see Figure 2.18). Reflex assessment and discussion of the specific reflexes can be found in Chapter 3.

Motor Output as a Reaction

Sherrill (1993) defines reactions as "automatic responses to sensory input that act to keep body parts in alignment, maintain equilibrium, and prevent injury" (p. 247). The reactions are influenced by cortical, basal ganglia, and cerebellar interaction. In typical development, reactions should appear between 2 to 18 months of development and remain throughout life (Milani-Comparetti, 1987; Milani-Comparetti & Gidoni, 1967). Reactions occur with normal muscle tone and the head and body's adjustment to the pull of gravity. Reactions should be facilitated through vestibular stimulation, equilibrium, and balance activities. Activities for developing balance may be reviewed in Chapter 9.

Motor Output as Skill

A motor skill is most often thought of as a motor action that an individual performs well. However, when working with infants or young children with disabilities, a motor skill may be achieved in a progressive pattern of development and may not be performed well or efficiently. Yet, the achievement of that skill may have taken months or years of repetition or practice. A meaningful definition of skill, especially when thinking of young or severely involved individuals, is selected from Cratty (1964), ". . . some learning has taken place or an integration of behavior has resulted" (p. 23).

FEEDBACK

Feedback is a term associated with learning a skill and is defined as the return of information or a part of the system output to its source so the output may be modified or improved. Infants and young children with delays or disabilities receive feedback from each sensory modality, but the most important is probably verbal feedback in the manner of praise from the teacher, caregiver, family member, or other children. Feedback serves as a source of motivation for the performer to continue practice of the motor skill or movement pattern (see Figure 2.19).

SUMMARY

This chapter provided a concise overview of the anatomy and function of the CNS. Most often, delay or disability involves the sensory or motor systems and it is necessary for the teacher, parent or caregiver to understand terminology associated with CNS dysfunction. In addition, the sensory systems were discussed in detail as part of the Perceptual Motor Response Theory Model. Often assessment outcomes are emphasized without a critical examination of sensory motor input or specific curricula activities.

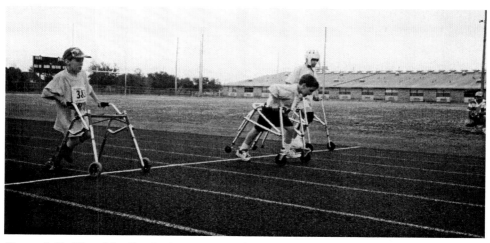

Figure 2.19. Visual feedback allows these young athletes to stay in their respective lanes as they participate in the GUMBO Classic.

REFERENCES

Auxter, D., Pyfer, J., & Huettig, C. (2005). *Principles and methods of adapted physical education and recreation.* Boston: McGraw-Hill.

Ayres, A. J. (1972). *Sensory integration and learning disorders.* Los Angeles: Western Psychological Services.

Ayres, A. J. (1978). Learning disabilities and the vestibular system. *Journal of Learning Disabilities, 11,* 18–29.

Ayres, A. J. (1989). *Sensory integration and praxis tests.* Los Angeles: Western Psychological Services.

Brodmann's cytoarchitectural map–Lateral view. (Adapted from Peele, R. L., 1954. The neuroanatomical basis for clinical neurology. New York: McGraw-Hill).

Brown, D. (1980). *Neurosciences for allied health therapies.* St. Louis, MO: C.V. Mosby.

Burt, A. (1993). *Textbook of neuroanatomy.* Philadelphia: WB. Saunders.

Cech, D., & Martin, S. (2002). *Functional movement development across a lifespan.* Philadelphia: WB. Saunders.

Coren, S., Ward, L., & Enns, J. T. (2004). *Sensation and perception* (6th ed.). Hoboken, NJ: Wiley & Sons.

Cratty, B. J. (1964). *Movement behavior and motor learning.* Philadelphia: Lea & Febiger.

DeGangi, G., & Greenspan, S. (1988). The development of sensory functions in infants. *Physical and Occupational Therapy in Pediatrics, 8*(4), 21–33.

Downey, J. A., & Darling, R. C. (Eds.). (1971). *Physiological basis of rehabilitation medicine.* Boston: Butterworth-Heinemann.

Dubowitz, L., Dubowitz, V., & Morante, A. (1980). Visual function in the newborn: A study of preterm and full-term infants. *Brain and Development, 2,* 15–27.

Eichstaedt, C. B., & Kalakian, L. H. (1993). *Developmental adapted physical education.* New York: Macmillan.

Ensher, G. L., & Clark, D. A. (1994). *Newborns at risk: Medical care and psychoeducational intervention* (2nd ed.). Gaithersburg, MD: Aspen.

Fenichel, G. M. (2005). *Clinical pediatric neurology* (5th ed.). Philadelphia: Elsevier/Saunders.

Fiorentino, M. R. (1963). *Reflex testing methods for evaluating C.N.S. development.* Springfield, IL: Charles C Thomas.

Fisher, A., Murray, E., & Bundy, A. (1991). *Sensory integration: Theory and practice.* Philadelphia: F.A. Davis.

Gallahue, D. L., & Ozmun, J. C. (2006). *Understanding motor development* (6th ed.) Boston: McGraw Hill.

Getman, G. (1952). *How to develop your child's intelligence: A research publication.* Luverne, MN: G.N. Getman.

Gonzalez, E. G., Myers, S. J., Downey, J. A., & Darling, R. C. (2001). *Downey & Darlings physiological basis of rehabilitative medicine.* Boston: Butterworth-Heinemann.

Haith, M. (1966). The response of the human newborn to visual movement. *Journal of Experimental Child Psychology, 3,* 235–243.

Hanson, M. J. (Ed.). (1996). *Atypical infant development* (2nd ed.). Austin, TX: Pro-Ed.

House, E. L., & Pansky, B. (1967). *A functional approach to neuroanatomy.* New York: McGraw-Hill.

Kolb, B., & Whishaw, I. Q. (2003). *Fundamentals of human neuropsychology* (5th ed.). New York: Worth.

Milani-Comparetti Motor Development Screening Test Manual (1987). Meyers Children's Rehabilitation Institute, University of Nebraska Medical Center, 444 South 44th Street, Omaha, NE 68131-3795.

Milani-Comparetti, A., & Gidoni, E. (1967). Pattern analysis of motor development and its disorders. *Developmental Medicine and Child Neurology, 9,* 625–630.

Morante, A., Dubowitz, L., Levene, M., & Dubowitz, V. (1982). The development of visual function in normal and neurologically abnormal preterm and full-term infants. *Developmental Medicine and Child Neurology, 24,* 771–784.

Noback, C. (2005). *The human nervous system: Structure and function.* Totowa, NJ: Humana Press.

Payne, V., & Isaacs, I. (2005). *Human motor development: A lifespan approach* (6th ed.). Boston: McGraw Hill.

Pederson, D., Evans, B., Chance, G., Bento, S., & Fox, A. (1988). Predictors of one-year developmental status in low birth weight infants. *Developmental and Behavioral Pediatrics, 9* (5), 287–292.

Peele, T. L. (1961). *The neuroanatomical basis for clinical neurology* (2nd ed.). New York: McGraw-Hill.

Reisman, J. (1987). Touch, motion, and proprioception. In P. Salapaatek & L. Cohen (Eds). *Handbook of infant perception, Vol 1: From sensation to perception* (pp. 265–303). Orlando, FL: Academic Press.

Rossetti, L. (1986). *High-risk infants: Identification, assessment, and intervention.* Austin, TX: Pro-Ed.

Royeen, C., & Lane, S. (1991). Tactile processing and sensory defensiveness. In A. G. Fisher, E. A. Murray, & A. C. Bundy. (Eds). *Sensory integration: Theory and practice* (pp. 108–136). Philadelphia: F.A. Davis.

Saigal, S., Szatmari, P., Rosenbaum, P., Campbell, D., & King, S. (1991). Cognitive abilities and school performance of extremely low birth weight children and matched term control children at age 8 years: A regional study. *Journal of Pediatrics, 118*(5), 751–760.

Seaman, J. A., & DePauw, K. P. (1995). *Sensory-motor experiences for the home: A manual for parents.* Reston, VA: American Association for Active Lifestyles and Fitness.

Sherrill, C. (1986). *Adapted physical education and recreation* (3rd ed.). Dubuque, IA: Wm. C. Brown.

Sherrill, C. (1993). *Adapted physical activity, recreation, and sport: Crossdisciplinary and lifespan* (4th ed.). Dubuque, IA: Brown and Benchmark.

Shumway-Cook, A., & Woollacott, M. H. (2001). *Motor control: Theory and practical applications* (2nd ed). Philadelphia: Williams & Wilkins.

Thompson, L., Fagan, J., & Fulker, D. (1991). Longitudinal prediction of specific cognitive abilities from infant novelty preference. *Child Development, 62,* 530–538.

Truex, R., & Carpenter, M. (1969). *Human neuroanatomy* (6th ed.). Baltimore: Williams & Wilkins.

Widerstrom, A., Mowder, B,. & Sandall, S. (1991). *At-risk and handicapped newborns and infants.* Englewood Cliffs, NJ: Prentice Hall.

Chapter 3

MUSCLE TONE

Chapter Objectives: After studying this chapter, the reader will be able to:
1. Discuss the importance of muscle tone in relation to assessment and intervention;
2. Discuss how abnormal muscle tone and primitive reflexes interfere with attaining developmental milestones;
3. List the observable signs of degrees of hypotonicity and hypertonicity;
4. Suggest principles to consider for proper positioning of infants and young children with hypertonocity;
5. List contraindicated actions or positions for children with hypertonic muscle tone.

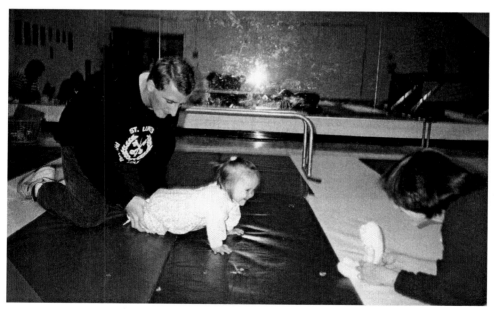

Figure 3.1. Increasing muscle tone allows the young girl to maintain this 4-point balance.

IMPORTANCE OF MUSCLE TONE

The single most important factor guiding assessment and intervention is an understanding of the importance of muscle tone. **Muscle tone** may be defined as contractile tension and readiness of muscles to perform movement. Two kinds of tone may be measured: (a) **phasic**, a rapid contraction in response to a high degree of stretch; and (b) **postural tone**, a prolonged contraction in response to a low-intensity stretch. Phasic tone is assessed by striking the patellar tendon to examine the quadriceps muscle contraction. Postural tone is measured by the ability of the infant to maintain position against gravity.

Infants who exhibit damage or diseases of the brain, spinal cord, nerves, and muscles may demonstrate hypotonia or hypertonia (Fenichel, 2005). Thelen (1986) stressed the importance of tonus control.

> Thus, at any point in development, the contribution of flexor or extensor, or right or left muscles may not be balanced. Since movement expression is a result of the relative dynamic balance between these agonist and antagonistic forces, the tonus of the muscles is one crucial determinant of the behavior pattern we observe, whatever the underlying pattern. (p. 113)

In addition, Bernstein (1967) emphasized the importance of muscle tonus by describing tonus in relation to coordination:

> It seems that there is at present evidence enough to decide upon a judgment, perhaps preliminary, and to say the following about tonus.
> (a) Tonus as an ongoing physiological adaptation and organization of the periphery is *not a condition of elasticity but a condition of readiness.*
> (b) Tonus is not merely a condition of the muscles but of the entire neuromuscular apparatus, including at least the final spinal synapse and the final common pathway.
> (c) Tonus, from this point of view, is related to coordination as a state is to an action or as a precondition is to an effect . . . not *a single case* of pathological coordination is known in which there is not at the same time a pathology of tonus, and that not a single central nervous apparatus is known which is related to one of these functions without being related to the other. (Bernstein, 1967, pp. 111–112)

Muscle tone is regulated by the cerebellar region of the brain which receives sensory impulses from the muscle spindles, golgi tendon organs, centers for vision, hearing, touch, and balance. Motor neurons primarily have two functions: (a) **excitation** or increasing muscle tension, and (b) **inhibition** or decreasing muscle tone. The identification of muscle tension from normal muscle tone is referred to as **hypotonia** (weak, floppy or decreased tone) or **hypertonia** (excessive spastic, or increased tone) (Rosenbaum, 1991; Sherrill, 2004). Observation of an infant or toddler during various states of arousal or responsivity often provides valuable insight regarding the child's degree of body tension.

Children with hypertonicity are usually identified most often due to association with damage to the major motor pathways of the brain which causes cerebral palsy (see Figure 3.2). **Spasticity** is a type of cerebral palsy resulting from lesions/damage to the pyramidal motor tract causing extreme muscle tension with various degrees of extensor and flexor hypertonicity. **Athetosis** is recognized by excessive, random movements and is caused by damage to the extrapyramidal nerve pathway which inhibits muscle tone. **Ataxic** cerebral palsy causes problems with balance, general incoordination, and abnormally low degrees of muscle tone.

Hypotonia has often been associated with mental delays, specifically infants with Down syndrome. However, there are numerous causes of hypotonia including genetic disorders, spinal cord disorders or injuries, spinal muscular atrophies, muscular dystrophies, and metabolic disorders. Low or weak muscle tone is characterized by flaccid muscles and poor body strength, balance and motor control. The **traction response** is the most often used method of assessing postural tone in a young child and is demonstrated by pulling the child by the arms to sitting and noting the amount of head lag and elbow flexion. A premature newborn of less than 33 weeks gestation will not demonstrate a traction response. Tendon reflexes would be absent or signifi-

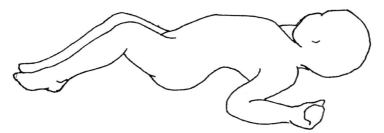

Figure 3.2. A child who demonstrates excessive hypertonicity may have cerebral hemisphere damage.

cantly depressed. If a child does not exhibit a traction response or has more than minimal head lag, it is abnormal hypotonia. Usually if the child has severe hypotonia and lacks sufficient strength for voluntary movement, the primitive reflexes will also not be strong (Fenichel, 2005). The "lying at rest position" of the infant can also be observed for hypotonia. If the child exhibits a "frog-leg" position with the arms lying limp or flaccid by the head, it is a clinical sign of hypotonia.

ASSESSMENT OF MUSCLE TONE AND REFLEXES

Most assessment instruments and intervention programs do not include methods for identifying the degrees of muscular weakness due to hypotonia. The following "Muscle Tone Index" (see Table 3.1) was developed to provide guidelines for assisting professionals with assessment of degrees of hypotonia versus hypertonia.

Table 3.1 Muscle Tone Index.

Definition: Contractile tension, resistance of muscles to stretch, or readiness to perform movements.

1. Extremes of Muscle Tone:
   Mushy like a "soft marshmallow," "limp like a doll," "hard as a rock," or "stiff as a board."
2. Firmness to Tactile Stimulation:
   Soft and flaccid—no solidity of the muscle.
   Slight feel of density or firmness.
   Series of movements cause slight increase of tension.
   Strong increase in muscular tone with movement.
   Uncontrollable movement of muscles (spasticity).
3. Resistance
   No resistance to active movement.
   Smooth flow of child initiated movements.
   Varied resistance of upper, lower or sides of body.
   Muscle firmness or tension increases with movement.
   Strong resistance to movement.
4. Ability to Maintain Posture:
   Control head, neck and trunk control.
   Extremities: upper, lower, left or right sides.
5. Support:
   Total teacher support to facilitate movement.
   Slight child support, but more teacher support.
   Child initiates movement; very little teacher facilitation.
   Child supports him/himself; no teacher support needed.

Assessment of excessive tone may often be observed by body positioning. If an infant or young child exhibits a tightly fisted hand enclosing the thumb with the fingers which does not open spontaneously, it is an indication of hypertonicity. In addition, if the positioning of the legs is adduction of the thighs with the legs and feet scissoring, this would be an indication of cerebral hemisphere dysfunction or spastic cerebral palsy. Assessment of primitive reflexes would be necessary (Fiorentino, 1963; Milani-Comparetti, 1987; Milani-Comparetti & Gidoni, 1967).

The development of motor patterns is dependent upon the suppression or integration of the following primitive reflexes into higher level and more refined movement actions and skills. Reflexes are involuntary movements which affect muscle tone, especially flexor and extensor tone, and are stimulated by changing the position of the head in relation to the body. Table 3.2 provides a detailed outline of each reflex with examples of the influence of primitive reflexes on motor development. The reflexes are considered normal for the time period listed; however, if they are assessed to be present after the given time period they may be an indicator of delayed maturation.

Table 3.2. Influence of Primitive Reflexes on Development of Motor Patterns.

Moro Reflex 0–4 mos.
Extension/flexion of limbs
Interferes with
-Use of arms for balance and use of
one arm at a time
-Protective extension & reactions
-Sitting position

Flexor Withdrawal 0–2 mos.
-Pressure to foot elicits a strong withdrawal of feet
-Interferes with standing & weight-bearing on feet

Crossed Extension 0–2 mos.
-Flexion of extended leg causes other leg to extend
-Interferes with crawling, creeping, standing, & walking

Asymetrical Tonic Neck 0–4 mos.
-Turning of the head to the side causes extension of the arm on the face side and flexion of the arm at the back of the head
-Interferes with rolling over and voluntary hand positioning, reaching, midline skills

continued

Table 3.2. Influence of Primitive Reflexes on Development of Motor Patterns—*Continued.*

Tonic Labyrinthine Supine 0–4 mos.
-In back lying position the child demonstrates increased extensor tone of extremities
-Interferes with raising of the head, bending of knees and reaching for feet, bringing of hands to midline

Hand Grasp Reflex 0–4 mos.
Wrapping of fingers around object placed in palm
Interferes with
-Voluntary grasp & release
-Weight-bearing with hands

Positive Supporting Reflex 3–8 mos.
-Holding the child in a standing position with soles of feet touching the floor the child's legs will demonstrate increased extensor tone
-Interferes with standing & walking
-May cause toe walking

Extensor Thrust 0–2 mos.
-Pressure to sole of foot elicits automatic and sudden leg extension
-Interferes with standing and later walking

Foot Grasp 0–9 mos.
-Deep pressure stimulation to bottom of feet causes toe flexion or clawing of toes
-Interferes with standing balance and walking

Symmetrical Tonic Neck 6–8 mos.
-Flexion of the head causes flexion of the arms and extension of the legs
-Extension or raising of the head causes arm extension & leg flexion (Bunny-hop)
-Interferes with creeping

Tonic Labyrinthine Prone 0–4 mos.
-When lying on the stomach the child demonstrates increased flexion
-Interferes with distal reach and lifting of head
-Interferes with extension of arms and legs

Activities for increasing muscle tone and strength may be referred to in Chapter 7. Activities for integration of primitive reflexes are located in Chapter 8.

POSITIONING AND HANDLING

Infants and young children with delays/disabilities may require assistance when moving from one position to another due to a muscle tone imbalance or lack of strength. Caregivers must initiate proper positioning and handling during all aspects of the child's daily routine including loading and unloading from transportation when arriving at child care, carrying, and feeding. To differentiate in terminology, **positioning** implies static movement of the child with assistance. **Handling** means to provide hands-on moving of the child from one place to another.

Improper positioning and handling can interfere with a child's progression in motor development. Simply carrying, handling, and positioning of young children can elicit and strengthen primitive reflex patterns which interfere with higher levels of functional mobility. A young child's caregivers should not adapt their positioning and handling techniques to the child's delayed or atypical reactions. Rather, caregivers must be aware of the child's muscle tone, equilibrium responses, and primitive reflex inhibition. Ultimately, the child should be allowed optimal independent movement, use of hands, and interaction with his/her peers. Therefore, it is imperative that all members of the interdisciplinary or cross-disciplinary team be knowledgeable of appropriate techniques of handling and positioning young children with hypertonic versus hypotonic motor development (Campbell, 1983; Scherzer & Tscharnuter 1990; Williamson, 1987). Team members (e.g., family, physical therapy, occupational therapy, speech therapy, education professionals) should collaborate regarding useful techniques for handling and positioning.

Techniques for proper positioning and handling are necessary for numerous reasons. The professional should always attempt to normalize muscle tone of children with hypertonicity and develop strength and endurance of children with low tone. Inhibition of abnormal primitive reflex activity, prevention of progressive secondary disabilities or deformities, and promotion of proper posture and body alignment are several reasons for providing guidance for essential physical growth and development. Health and respiratory problems are common with infants and young children and proper positioning improves cardiorespiratory efficiency. In addition, providing the child with a sense of security and stability enhances the child's ability to organize sensory-motor information (Campbell, 1983; Diamant, 1992; Finnie, 1997; Fiorentino, 1963, 1981; Levitt, 2003, Parks, 1992; Scherzer & Tscharnuter, 1990; Sherrill, 2004).

Guidelines for Positioning and Handling

The caregiver should implement the following guidelines when positioning and handling a child with muscle tone imbalance:

- Prepare the child for interaction by telling him/her what will be done before and throughout movements.
- A soft, low spoken tone of voice will forewarn the child of the forthcoming touch or positioning—and prevent startling responses, especially of a child with hypertonicity.
- Gentle rocking or massaging and slow rotational, flexor, and extensor movements of the extremities will assist with relaxing children with hypertonicity.
- Children with hypotonicity will need a more upbeat and exciting approach to ready them for exercise periods.
- Always guide a child through a movement pattern or change positions slowly allowing her to complete as many movements as possible.
- Provide support to the involved joints never allowing joints to go beyond normal ranges of motion. Do not pull a child into a position by placing your hands on his distal joints.
- Remember changes in head position will initiate primitive reflex patterns (see Figure 3.3). Children with spasticity will demonstrate asymmetrical tonic neck reflex patterns and increased extensor tone when in the back lying position. In the 4-point position raising of the head will cause extension of the arms and flexion or bending of the hips, knees, and ankles (i.e., "Bunny-hop").
- Decrease abnormal muscle tone and attempt to normalize typical posture and movement patterns.
- If a child demonstrates increased extensor tone in the extremities, position him so that the opposite pattern of flexion is achieved. By following this principle, the tight or contracted muscles will be stretched or relaxed and the opposite muscles will be strengthened.
- When positioning the child in supine be sure the head and arms are in midline as turning of the head to the side will initiate the asymmetrical tonic neck reflex. The child may need to have slight support (e.g., a small wedge or pillow) under his head, shoulders, and trunk. The hips should be flexed slightly with the legs separated, abducted, and flexed slightly.

- When positioning the child in prone, the hips and legs should be extended and abducted slightly. Place a small wedge or pillow under the child's chest to assist in lifting the chest and bearing weight on the upper extremities. Place the child's elbows slightly below the shoulders. Encourage the child to alternate between weight-bearing on the elbows and hands. Encourage upper extremity extension by placing a toy within the child's forward reach.
- Side-lying is considered a neutral position for decreasing reflex patterns and increasing postural organization. The child's body is extended on the weight-bearing side and flexed on the non-weight-bearing side.

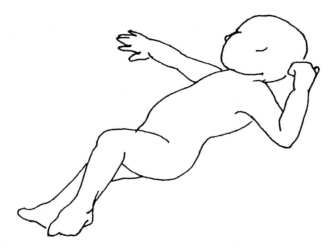

Figure 3.3. Turning of the head sideward initiates the asymmetrical tonic neck reflex.

- Supports such as a pillow (or bag of sugar or flour) can be placed alongside the child and between the child's legs to help her maintain the position. The child should not be placed in the position beyond which length of time the predominant primitive reflexes pull her out of the side-lying position.
- When positioning the child in sitting, be sure her hips, knees, and ankles are securely placed at 90 degree angles (see Figures 3.4 and 3.5). The child's weight should be on his pelvis, not his trunk. His head should be in midline and flexed slightly. You may need to use wedges, bolsters, or rolled towels to assist the child with maintain-

ing the position. Provide footrests when using chairs. Baby jumpers and walkers often do not provide sufficient support to promote proper tone and posture. In addition, they may allow the child's hips to be externally rotated for extended periods of time (a contraindicated position for a child with joint laxity).

• Do not allow a child with hypotonicity or hypertonicity to sit for lengthy periods of time in the "W" position (see Figure 3.6). Although this position provides the child stability, it stresses the muscles, joints, and ligaments and does not allow for the use of equilibrium and righting reactions.

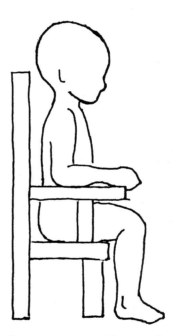

Figure 3.4. This child is securely supported and balanced while sitting with the hips, knees, and ankles at 90 degree angles.

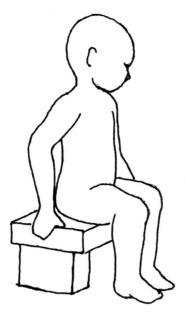

Figure 3.5. As the child gains muscle tone and strength back and arm support can be reduced or removed from the chair.

- In supported standing, align the child's trunk over the base of support. Encourage the child to stand upright with the pelvis and hip forward. The child's feet should be flat and separated to shoulder width apart with the toes pointing forward. Position the child close to the support surface to assist with maintaining this alignment and weight distribution. The child should be encouraged to shift her weight to reach all directions for a toy.
- A child should not be left in a position for lengthy periods of time. Always provide the child with an engaging activity during the time the child is maintaining a desired position. Alternate the child's position frequently. Remember the child's head should be placed in midline and arms brought forward to facilitate interaction with a toy or other object (Campbell, 1983; Diamant, 1992; Finnie, 1997; Fiorentino, 1963, 1981; Johnson-Martin, Jens, Attermeier, & Hacker, 1991; Levitt, 2003; Parks, 2006; Scherzer & Tscharnuter, 1990; Sherrill, 1993).

Carrying

The guidelines given below should be followed when carrying a child with muscle tone imbalance. In addition, some of the positions can be used during individualized warm-up routines of stretching or relaxing the muscles (Coling, 1991; Finnie, 1997; Scherzer & Tscharnuter, 1990). Carrying the child so she faces forward provides an opportunity for her to interact with the environment. Figure 3.7 depicts proper positioning and handling when carrying a child with predominate extensor muscle tone.

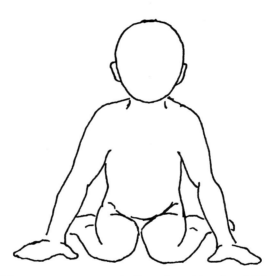

Figure 3.6. The "W" position is a contraindicated position for children with hypertonicity and hypotonicity.

- Tuck the child's head down and provide support at the back of the head and neck. Bring the child's arms forward. The caregiver can separate the lower extremities by placing her hands between the child's legs (see Figure 3.8).

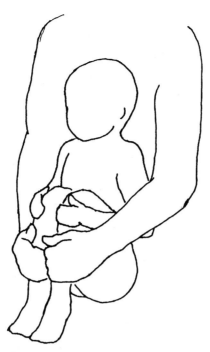

Figure 3.7. A child with predominate extensor tone should be carried in a flexed position. Depending on the child's body weight, the caregiver may need to place one arm under the child's legs for support.

- Carry the child lower (in relation to your body) to provide more support to his head and trunk; carry him higher to encourage him to exhibit independent head, neck, and trunk control. Alternate carrying the child on both sides of your body to promote symmetry of the trunk and pelvis.
- Do not straddle a child with joint laxity across your hips. Carry the child in front of your trunk (see Figure 3.9).

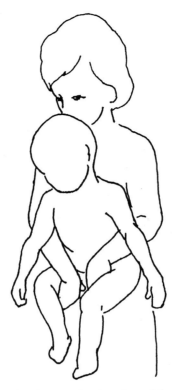

Figure 3.8. To break-up excessive tone and scissoring of the legs and feet, the caregiver's arms or hands can be placed between the child's lower extremities.

- One way to carry a child with hypotonicity or hypertonicity is to seat the child across one of your arms with her hips and knees at 90 degree angles; use your shoulder or chest to support the child's head and trunk. To break up the tone of the child with hypertonicity, flex or elevate one leg.
- A child with low tone can also be carried in prone or supine over your arms. The prone position will encourage extension against gravity. If scissoring of the lower extremities is present, separate the lower extremities with your arm. Place your hand on the child's trunk or shoulders. Encourage the child to lift his head (see Figures 3.10 and 3.11).

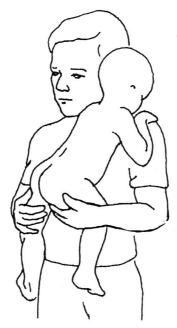

Figure 3.9. Carry a child with joint laxity in front of your trunk while supporting the hips. This position also helps decrease the hypertonicity and scissoring of the lower extremities in a child with spasticity.

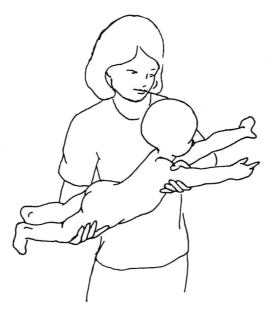

Figure 3.10. While carrying the child with hypotonicity in the prone position, provide elongation of the extremities and encourage lifting of the head.

- To decrease the scissoring or flexion of a child with hypertonicity, carry her in a side-lying position with your arm separating her legs and, if necessary, bending one knee higher than the other; use your hand to cross the child's trunk and support the arms and head (see Figure 3.12). This position also encourages lateral righting of the head and trunk.

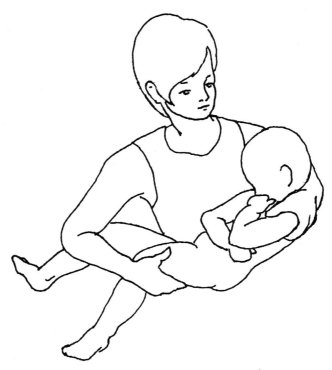

Figure 3.11. Bending the hips of the child with hypertonicity (e.g., spasticity) prior to lifting him will help to decrease the tone in the lower extremities and allow you to carry the child in a flexed position.

- When using infant carriers, car seats, or strollers:
  - choose ones with solid seats and backs; provide side supports if necessary;
  - provide proximal support with towels, pillows, small wedges, etc.;
  - bring the child's arms forward and use small rolls to properly align his legs.

Feeding

The following guidelines are suggested for feeding a child with a delay/disability (Coling, 1991; Finnie, 1997; Morris & Klein, 2000; Poulton & Sexton, 1995; Williamson, 1987). Team members should communicate regarding each child's specific needs.

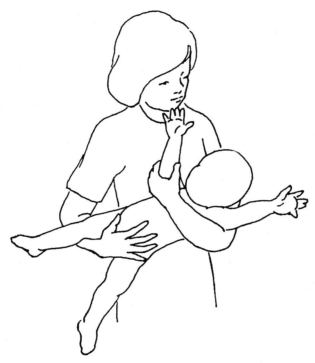

Figure 3.12. The flexion or scissoring of the extremities by a child with hypertonicity can be decreased by carrying the child with the extremities extended.

- Always place the child in an upright or half-upright position during feeding. Never allow the child to drink from a bottle or cup while in a lying position.
- Provide the child with proximal support and bring her arms forward so she can practice self-feeding skills. Be sure her feet are supported on a flat surface.
- Provide oral relaxation or stimulation as needed.
- Hold the nipple/spoon below the child's mouth and slightly away

from the child to encourage the child to come forward.
- Assist the child in holding the bottle/cup with two hands.
- Keep the child in an upright position for 30 minutes after eating.

Lifting

In order to protect yourself and the child from injuries, proper lifting strategies, such as the ones given below, should be employed each time you lift a child to position, handle, or carry her (Finnie, 1997; Lasko & Knopf, 1984; Scull, 1996).

- Do not lift (without assistance) a child who weighs more than 35 percent of your body weight.
- Prior to lifting, analyze the child's muscle tone, reflex involvement, current position, and desired position.
- Before lifting the child, place her close to your center of gravity. Scoop her into your body to provide support and stability to her joints and extremities. If the child is in prone or supine, roll her over into side-lying before lifting her to prevent initiation of primitive reflexes. Separate your feet and place one foot ahead of the other. Tighten your stomach muscles just prior to lifting.
- During lifting, keep your back straight and bend your knees. Do not twist your trunk while holding a child; move your feet to turn.
- To pick a child up from a low surface, kneel close to the child. Never bend over from standing to pick up a child.
- To lower a child from a carrying position to a low surface, bend to your knees keeping your back straight as you kneel, then transfer the child. Never bend over from standing to lower a child.
- If transferring a child to a chair, be certain the chair is stable and remove any straps or seat belts from the center of the chair.
- If you are standing for a lengthy duration while holding a child, decrease the strain on your back by lifting one of your feet onto a low surface (e.g., stool, step, curb).

SUMMARY

The influence of muscle tone and primitive reflexes must be understood in relation to pediatric assessment and intervention. Proper use of positioning and handling techniques reinforces desirable developmental outcomes. In addition to prescribing an individualized pediatric developmental motor intervention, professionals should provide caregivers with suggestions for relaxation, sensory stimulation, and appropriate positioning and handling of their child.

REFERENCES

Bernstein, N. A. (1967). *The coordination and regulation of movements.* New York: Pergamon Press.

Campbell, P. (1983). *Introduction to neurodevelopmental treatment.* Akron, OH: Children's Hospital Medical Center of Akron.

Coling, M. C. (1991). *Developing integrated programs: A transdisciplinary approach for early intervention.* Tucson, AZ: Therapy Skill Builders.

Diamant, R. B. (1992). *Positioning for play: Home activities for parents of young children.* Tucson, AZ: Communication Skill Builders.

Fenichel, G. M. (2005). *Clinical pediatric neurology: A signs and symptoms approach* (5th ed.). Philadelphia: Elsevier/Saunders.

Finnie, N. R. (1997). *Handling the young cerebral palsied child at home* (3rd ed.). Boston: Butterworth-Heinemann.

Fiorentino, M. (1963). *Reflex testing methods for evaluating C.N.S. development.* Springfield, IL: Charles C Thomas.

Fiorentino, M. (1981). *A basis for sensorimotor development: Normal and abnormal.* Springfield, IL: Charles C Thomas.

Johnson-Martin, N. M., Jens, K. G., Attermeier, S. M., & Hacker, B. J. (1991). *The Carolina curriculum for infants and toddlers with special needs* (2nd ed.). Baltimore: Paul H. Brookes.

Lasko, P. M., & Knopf, K. G. (1984). *Adapted and corrective exercise for the disabled adult.* Dubuque, IA: Eddie Bowers.

Levitt, S. (2003). *Treatment of cerebral palsy and motor delay* (4th ed.). Palo Alto, CA: Blackwell Scientific Publications.

Milani-Comparetti Motor Development Screening Test Manual. (1987). Meyers Children's Rehabilitation Institute, University of Nebraska Medical Center, 444 South 44th Street, Omaha, NE 68131-3795.

Milani-Comparetti, A., & Gidoni, E. (1967). Pattern analysis of motor development and its disorders. *Developmental Medicine and Child Neurology, 9,* 625–630.

Morris, S. E., & Klein, M. D. (2000). *Pre-feeding skills: A comprehensive resource for feeding development* (2nd ed.). Tucson, AZ: Therapy Skill Builders.

Parks, S. (2006). *Inside help.* Palo Alto, CA: VORT

Poulton, S., & Sexton, D. (1995). Feeding young children: Developmentally appropriate considerations for supplementing family care. *Childhood Education, 72* (2), p. 66–71.

Rosenbaum, D. A. (1991). *Human motor control.* San Diego, CA: Academic Press.

Scherzer, A. L., & Tscharnuter, I. (1990). *Early diagnosis and therapy in cerebral palsy: A primer on infant developmental problems* (2nd ed. rev. expanded). New York: Marcel

Dekker.

Scull, S. A. (1996). Mobility and ambulation. In L. A. Kurtz, P. W. Dowrick, S. E. Levy, & M. L. Batshaw (Eds.), *Handbook of Developmental Disabilities: Resources for Interdisciplinary Care* (pp. 269–326). Gaithersburg, MD: Aspen.

Sherrill, C. (1993). *Adapted physical activity, recreation, and sport: Crossdisciplinary and lifespan* (4th ed.). Dubuque, IA: Brown & Benchmark.

Sherrill, C. (2004). *Adapted physical activity, recreation, and sport: Crossdisciplinary and lifespan* (6th ed.). New York: McGraw Hill.

Thelen, E. (1986). Development of coordinated movement: Implications for early human development. In M. G. Wade & H. T. A. Whiting (Eds.), *Motor Development in Children: Aspects of Coordination and Control* (pp. 107–124). Dordrecht, Netherlands: Martinus Nijhoff.

Williamson, G. G. (1987). *Children with spina bifida: Early intervention and preschool programming*. Baltimore: Paul H. Brookes.

Chapter 4

MEDICAL AND BIOLOGICAL CONSIDERATIONS

Chapter Objectives:
1. Demonstrate knowledge of definitions and criteria for eligibility for receiving early intervention services according to Part C of IDEA;
2. Identify complications of prematurity and low birth weight that may hinder normal infant/toddler development;
3. Gain an understanding of physical and mental conditions that may result in developmental delay;
4. Understand terminology associated with medical procedures and diagnosis;
5. Engage in knowledgeable conversation with a child's caregivers concerning medical issues;
6. Identify and distinguish the disorders included in the category of Pervasive Developmental Disorder;
7. Understand autism spectrum disorders and the impact on the developing child;
8. Identify the effects of autism spectrum disorders on sensory dysfunction and discuss intervention by the movement specialist;
9. Discuss the value of teaming when working with young children with medical conditions.

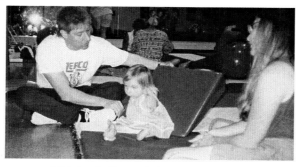

Figure 4.1. This young child is challenged from a congenital anomaly and is totally dependent on trunk strength to sit and maintain upright posture.

This chapter provides a brief summary of the disabilities that have been adopted by states to determine eligibility for early intervention services in accord with The Individuals with Disabilities Education Improvement Act, (IDEA), Public Law 108-446 (Section 634) (December, 2004). Part C of IDEA includes infants and toddlers, ages birth through two years inclusive (36) months and their families. The criteria for eligibility have not been changed in the newest reauthorization of IDEA, and include infants and toddlers with developmental delay or a diagnosed physical or mental condition that has a high risk for developmental delay.

The chapter begins with a brief discussion of factors that occur before and after birth that by themselves are not determining factors for eligibility to receive Part C services. However, when several conditions occur at the same time and are due to the same set of circumstances, an infant may experience developmental delays that become significant.

PREMATURITY AND LOW BIRTH WEIGHT

Major issues which cause trauma for infants are prematurity and low birth weight. A full-term infant is considered to be between 37 and 41 weeks gestation; therefore, a premature infant is less than 37 weeks gestation or below birth weight of 2,500 grams (approx. 5.5 lbs.) (Howard, Williams, Port, & Lepper, 1997; Koller, Lawson, Rose, Wallace, & McCarton, 1997; McCarton, Wallace, Divon, & Vaughan, 1996). Very low birth weight (VLBW) is less than 1,500 grams (3 lb. 5 oz.) and extremely low birth weight is 750 grams (1 lb. 10 oz). Survival rates of infants with low birth weight and prematurity have increased greatly over the past 15 years (see Figure 4.2). Technology and improved medical management have made it possible for infants as young as 23-weeks gestation (micropremature infants) to survive; however, these children will have a strong probability for many medical complications. Health factors for premature infants improve as the period of gestation increases. Research associates early neurological abnormalities with later cognitive outcomes (Koller et al., 1997; McCarton et al., 1996).

Medical complications that may occur as a result of prematurity and low birth weight include hypoxia, apnea, ischemic encephalopathy, intraventricular hemorrhage, respiratory distress, bronchopulmonary dysplasia, and hyperbilirubinemia. Premature newborns with low birth weight will require Level III neonatal intensive care facilities. Hospitals are rated as Level I (community hospital, low numbers of infants delivered, and very little technological equipment for handling major risk factors), Level II (facility that can manage a large number of deliveries, but only select mothers and newborns with minor complications) and Level III (facility with "state of art" equipment and specialists for taking care of mother and newborn with high risk factors and needing neonatal intensive care units) (Ensher & Clark, 1994).

The following are definitions of frequently occurring conditions of gestation, delivery, and neonatal period:

Premature Labor. Contractions of the uterus and cervical dilation occur prior to 37 weeks of gestation. Prematurity may be caused by stress, nutrition, age, prenatal exposure to drugs (alcohol, cocaine/crack, marijuana, and methamphetamines), cigarette smoking, chronic diseases (hypertension, cardiovascular disease, diabetes), infectious diseases, and other factors.

Placenta Previa. A fertilized egg is introduced in the bottom of the uterus instead of the top of the uterus causing the placenta to implant and cover the opening of the cervix. Maternal bleeding can occur and may be a large amount in a short period of time causing trauma to the mother and high occurrence for loss of the unborn infant.

Abruptio Placenta. This condition involves varying degrees of separation of the placenta from the wall of the uterus which interferes with the crucial functions of the placenta. The placenta functions are to provide oxygen and nutrients and eliminate waste products.

Amniotic Fluid and Premature Rupture of Membranes. One of the most important roles of the amniotic fluid is to serve as a shock absorber in a temperature-controlled and gravity-free environment for the fetus. If the membrane surrounding the infant breaks prematurely, early delivery puts the infant at high risk for infection and other problems associated with premature delivery and increased risk for trauma. Factors which may cause a premature rupture of membranes and loss of fluids may include stress, fetal movements, nutrition, and exposure to teratogens.

Entangled Umbilical Cord. The umbilical cord contains all nutrients and oxygenated blood from the fetus side of the placenta and connects to the fetus. In normal circumstances the cord is cut upon delivery and is shed by the infant within 7–10 days after birth. Under some circumstances the infant becomes wrapped in the cord causing decreased blood supply to the infant and possible asphyxiation. Monitoring equipment provides information that assists with determining the amount of time the infant may have had limited oxygen supply. A lack of oxygen may cause neurological damage.

Meconium Aspiration Syndrome. Meconium is an accumulation of feces in the bowel of the fetus. The muscles of the infant's rectum should not relax until after birth. However, due to difficulties during delivery the infant's mouth and nose may contain amniotic fluid with meconium and other fetal waste products. The infant may have had decreased oxygen or asphyxia during delivery causing the infant to wheeze for air. Abnormalities that may occur from meconium aspiration syndrome may affect the infant's neurological, cardiovascular, and respiratory systems. The infant with this syndrome is at high risk for neurological problems and chronic lung disease including aspiration pneumonia (Batshaw, 2002; Blackman, 1997; Ensher & Clark, 1994; Howard et al., 1997).

Hyperbilirubinemia. Infants born prematurely and with low birth weight may have an increased amount of bilirubin (a yellow pigment) resulting from a breakdown of red blood cells in the liver. For those infants who survive the resulting abnormalities may include cerebral palsy, high-frequency hearing loss, discoloration of teeth, and visual impairments. This clinical syndrome is known as **kernicterus** (Batshaw, 2002).

Apgar. In 1953, Virginia Apgar, an anesthesiologist, devised a rating system of the newborn infant's physiological status at birth. The Apgar Score (Apgar, 1953), determined at one and five minutes after birth, remains a widely-used method of assessing the infant's health, development, responsivity, and adaptation to extrauterine life. The 1-minute score describes the intrauterine distress level the infant experienced. The 5-minute score is indicative of morbidity and mortality. The infant is given a score of "0", "1", or "2" for the following five parameters: activity (muscle tone), pulse (heart rate), grimace (reflex, irritability), appearance (color), and respiration. A "0" denotes no response for that parameter. A "1" denotes a transitional score between "0" and "2". A "2" denotes the best response for that parameter. Thus, the infant could receive an overall score between 0 and 10 at either assessment. If the overall score is 6 or less the infant may be

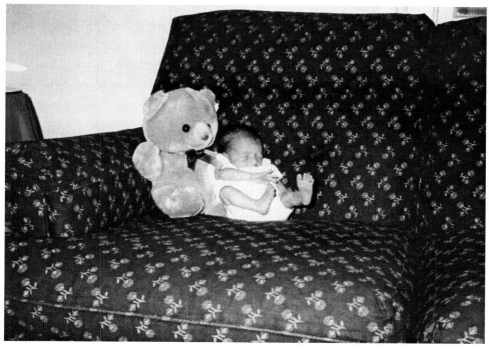

Figure 4.2. Medical management has greatly improved the developmental outcomes of a premature and low-birth weight baby.

medically at-risk (Blackman, 1997; Ensher & Clark, 1994; Widerstrom, Mowder, & Sandall, 1991).

MEDICAL CONDITIONS

Physical and mental conditions of newborns and infants have a high probability of resulting in developmental delay. They include genetic variations (e.g., chromosomal abnormalities, single gene defects, anomalies of unknown etiologies), congenital infections, sensory impairments, orthopedic and neurologic conditions, hemorrhage, technology dependence, drug exposure and psychiatric disturbance. The more frequently occurring conditions are discussed in this chapter.

Genetic Variations

We ought not to set them aside with idle thoughts or idle words about "curiosities" or "chances." Not one of them is without meaning; not one that might not

become the beginning of excellent knowledge, if only we could answer the
question—why is it rare or being rare, why did it in this instance happen?
(James Paget, 1882, as cited in Jones, 1997, p. 1)

It is critically important for professionals to have a basic understanding of the various patterns of genetic malformations and develop
practical applications for early intervention based on the unique needs
of each child. Often caregivers will consult with the dysmorphologist
or geneticist who has assisted with identifying the etiology, prognosis,
and plan of management for the child. This section will provide information regarding the more common genetic variations or malformations occurring during the process of human development.

Chromosomes are the basic genetic units of the human being and
each chromosome consists of hundreds of genes. In fact, approximately 100,000 genes (which are in pairs) compose the human being
(Jones, 1997). A chromosome is a chain of deoxyribonucleic acid
(DNA). Each gene has a particular location on the chromosome. In
each human cell there are 23 pairs of chromosomes (46 chromosomes), one pair from the father and one pair from the mother.
Twenty-two pairs, called **autosomes** are identical in males and
females. The 23rd pair of chromosomes is termed the **sex chromosome** which determines the child's gender. The sex chromosomes
consists of two X chromosomes in the female and an X and Y chromosome in the male. The mother can only contribute an X chromosome; therefore, the child's sex is determined by the father.

Normal development is dependent on gene content and gene balance of chromosomes. During cell division an altered number of chromosomes may occur which in turn cause faulty chromosome distribution. During the gametic (gametes—sex cells) meiotic reduction division, one of each pair of autosomes and one of the sex chromosomes
are distributed randomly to each daughter cell (cells to-be have one
chromsome from each pair—23 chromosomes). During mitosis, each
replicated chromosome is pulled apart longitudinally at the centromere so that each daughter cell has identical chromosome complements (46 chromosomes) (Jones, 1997). Faulty chromosome distribution is not completely understood; however, one recognized factor is
the increasing age of the mother. Genetic disorders are also caused in
part by a mutation in the chemical coding (DNA) of a single gene or
gene pair. A mutation can occur by chance or as a result of external

factors such as drugs, virus, or radiation. Children born with genetic variations (as determined by a licensed medical doctor) include but are not restricted to conditions within the categories of chromosome abnormalities, single gene defects, and anomalies of unknown etiologies.

Chromosomal Abnormalities

The correct number of chromosomes in humans is 46, a number which remains constant. Chromosomal rearrangements and variations in the number of chromosomes result in congenital malformations which involve hundreds of genes. Diagnosis of abnormality is completed through a process termed karotyping.

Down Syndrome. Down syndrome, Trisomy 21, was first identified in 1866 by Langdon Down and is one of the leading causes of mental retardation (Howard et al., 1997). Down syndrome is caused by one of three types of chromosomal defects: nondisjunction (most common), mosaicism, and translocation. Trisomy 21 is typically associated with nondisjunction, whereby there is an error in cell division of the egg or sperm prior to fertilization. Instead of the normal 46 chromosomes (23 pair), individuals with Trisomy 21 have an extra 21st chromosome due to failure of the 21st chromosome pair to separate. This results in a total of 47 chromosomes instead of the normal 46 (Cohen, 1996). Nondisjunction usually occurs sporadically and recurs at a rate of .5 to 1 percent (Blackman, 1997).

In mosaicism, abnormal separation of the chromosome occurs after fertilization in the second or third division of the embryo. Only a portion of cells have the extra 21st chromosome (47), while many cells have the typical number (46). The rate of recurrence is not different from the general population (Blackman, 1997). In translocation, misguided genetic material (all or a part of one chromosome) becomes attached to another chromosome during cell division. "Approximately half of the time, this type of Down syndrome is inherited from a parent who is a carrier" (Blackman, 1997, p. 98–99). Therefore, there is a greater risk of recurrence than with other types of Down syndrome. Different causes of Down syndrome are associated with different developmental outcomes and physical characteristics. Children with the mosaic or translocation form of Down syndrome may have fewer physical traits and greater intellectual potential (Fishler & Koch, 1991);

however, research has been controversial (Johnson & Abelson, 1969; Vaughn & Goldberg, 1994).

Diagnostic indicators of Down syndrome include hypotonia, joint laxity, short stature, flat facial profile, slanted palpebral fissures, abnormal external ears, mental retardation, poor balance, and congenital heart and inner ear problems (American Academy of Pediatrics Committee on Genetics, 1994) (see Figure 4.3). Fifty percent of infants with Down syndrome may have congenital heart disease; however, there is no current scientific knowledge to clearly support the frequency of other congenital problems. There is an increased frequency of thyroid dysfunction in infants with Down syndrome, but presently there are no recommendations by the Down Syndrome Medical Interest Group (DSMIG) for appropriate frequency or adequacy of the thyroid examination (Cohen, 1996).

In addition, families of infants with Down syndrome should utilize the growth and head circumference charts specifically developed for this population. A child who is not developing according to this devel-

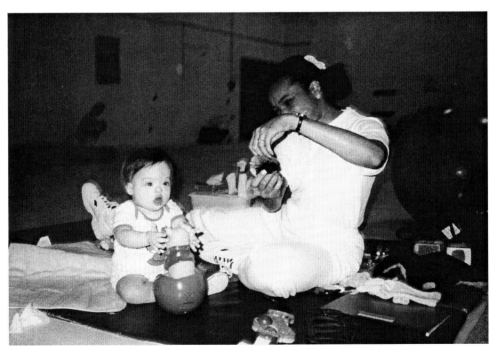

Figure 4.3. Infants with Down syndrome should be provided interventions in gross motor and visual motor coordination.

opmental growth chart should be checked for possible thyroid, pituitary, congenital heart, or nutritional disorders (Cohen, 1996).

Turner Syndrome. Also known as XO syndrome, this syndrome is found only in females and is a sex chromosome abnormality that occurs when one of the two X chromosomes is absent or partially absent. Abnormalities include extremely small stature and tendency for obesity, immature development of reproductive organs, webbing of fingers or toes, extra skin of the neck, kidney and cardiovascular problems, and congenital edema of the extremities at birth (Garron, 1977; Jones, 1997; Thompson, 1989). There is usually much delay in motor skills and poor coordination. It is reported that the average IQ for most individuals with Turner Syndrome ranges from 90–95 with a specific pattern of learning disabilities, including visual memory problems effecting reading and mathematical abilities (Howard et al., 1997).

Fragile X Syndrome. The genetic abnormality Fragile X (also known as Martin-Bell Syndrome and Marker X Syndrome) is considered to be the leading known cause of mental retardation, although professionals report to be more knowledgeable of Down syndrome. Mental retardation is more prevalent in males. Fifty percent of females with Fragile X have mental delays and educational difficulties (Jones, 1997). Infants have a normal appearance at birth although later features of males include a prominent forehead, jaw and chin; large bat ears; and enlarged testicles. Females exhibit less distinctive features. Individuals exhibit behavioral problems and specific autistic-like characteristics including hand flapping, biting, and rocking. Verbal and language disorders include perseveration, echolalia, and bizarre or inappropriate speech responses. "Cluttering," an abnormal speech pattern, occurs in individuals with higher intelligence levels (Jones, 1997). Motor skills are delayed in early childhood (American Academy of Pediatrics Committee on Genetics, 1994; Dykens, Hodapp, Ort, & Leckman, 1993; Kurtz, Dowrick, Levy, & Batshaw, 1996; Santos, 1992).

Single Gene Defects

Single gene defects may involve one or both genes of a chromosome pair. Four types of gene disorders include **autosomal dominant, autosomal recessive, X-linked dominant** and **X-linked**

recessive. Autosomal dominant disorders are caused by an alteration in a single gene along one of the autosomes. If only one parent should carry the gene, there is a 50:50 chance of passing the defect to the offspring with each pregnancy. However, if both parents are affected, there is a 75 percent risk that each child will inherit the disorder. Autosomal recessive disorders are less likely to manifest a disorder and both parents must pass the affected gene to the child. X-linked recessive disorders occur more frequently in the male population than female population (Pueschel, 1978; Widerstrom et al., 1991).

Phenylketonuria (PKU). PKU is an inherited autosomal recessive inborn error of amino acid metabolism. The child's system does not produce a necessary liver enzyme therefore allowing the amino acid, phenylalanine, to build up in the blood stream until it becomes toxic. Screening is usually done in all newborns because the disorder cannot be detected by prenatal amniocentesis. If untreated, progressive brain damage will result, including defective myelination, microcephaly, mental retardation, seizures, hyperactivity, and poor physical growth. A diet low in phenylalanine (meat, milk, dairy products) and vitamin supplements may reduce further delays. Lofenalac formula and Phenyl-Free (food source for older children) are the most often-used products. It is unclear if dietary restrictions may be lifted later in life, but it becomes much harder for the family to maintain an age-appropriate diet and control the older child's eating habits (Howard et al., 1997; Kurtz et al., 1996).

Hypothyroidism. This genetic condition is an autosomal recessive metabolic disorder in which there is a disorder of thyroid hormone production causing the infant to be small, hypotonic, and severely mentally retarded. Screening procedures initiated in the early 1970s proved to be effective in detecting hypothyroidism; however, when a prior family history is not known, perinatal screening may not be performed. Symptoms of a newborn may include abnormal facial features (broad, flat nose and widely-set eyes), hypotonia, enlarged tongue, and lethargy. Combined with current treatments and early intervention, the child may progress in school at higher levels, but will still exhibit delay of motor skills, visual motor perception, and speech and language (Howard et al., 1997; Kurtz et al., 1996; Peterson, 1987).

Tuberous Sclerosis. This syndrome, an autosomal dominant or sporadic disorder, is visually obvious due to an unusual "butterfly" rash on the infant's face. Characteristics include seizures, mental retardation, adenoma sebaceum (tumorous skin glands), calcium deposits in the brain, malignancies, hydrocephalus and tumors of the heart (Howard et al., 1997; Kwiatkowski & Short, 1994; Kurtz et al., 1996). Treatment for seizures is utilized.

Abnormalities or Syndromes of Unknown Etiology

Spina Bifida. Spina bifida is a congenital defect of the central nervous system and is defined as a cleft spine that involves incomplete closure in the spinal column. The condition is nonprogressive and there is no cure for spina bifida because the nerve tissue cannot be replaced or repaired. The term spina bifida is of Latin origin and means "split" or "open" spine. Spina bifida occurs between the 4th–6th week of pregnancy, whereby two sides of the embryo's spine fail to join together and leaves an open area. Spina bifida occurs in about 1 per 1000 live births and is the second leading cause of orthopedic conditions in school age children (Sherrill, 2004). Although the exact cause is unknown, it does appear to run in families. The risk of having a second child with spina bifida is approximately 3–4 percent.

It is possible to detect spina bifida and other neural tube defects prenatally by testing the mother's blood for alpha-fetoprotein (AFP) during the 18th week of pregnancy. This measures the amount of AFP that the fetus is producing. Doctors also use ultrasound to see if a baby has spina bifida, as the spinal defect can be seen on the ultrasound. Maternal folic acid deficiency has also been linked to spina bifida. Folic acid consumption by the mother is highly recommended and can be found in orange juice, dark green leafy vegetables, eggs, and many multivitamins.

There are two forms of spina bifida: spina bifida occulta and spina bifida manifesta. Spina bifida manifesta includes meningocele and myelomeningocele (Nemours Foundation, 2006). These three types of spina bifida (occulta, meningocele, and myelomeningocele) vary from mild to severe. Myelomeningocele (MM) is the most common and severe form of spina bifida, whereby the spinal cord and nerve roots exit between vertebrae and form in a sac outside the body. Surgery is usually performed during the first 24 hours after birth typically to push the spine back into the vertebral column. This procedure closes the hole to protect the spinal cord and prevent infection. However, the effects may be moderate to severe and may include muscle weakness or paralysis below the area of the spine where the incomplete closure (cleft) occurs, loss of sensation below the cleft, and loss of bowel and bladder control. In addition to physical and mobility difficulties, most individuals have some form of learning disabilities. Some children may have attention deficit hyperactivity disorder (ADHD) and learning disabilities including hand-eye coordination problems.

Most babies who are born with MM spina bifida also have hydrocephalus, an accumulation of fluid in and around the brain. A baby with hydrocephalus must have a shunt (thin tube) placed in the brain to relieve pressure on the brain by draining and diverting the increase of fluid. Some children will need subsequent surgeries to manage the shunt, spine, feet, and hips. Many children with MM spina bifida must learn to manage bowel and bladder functions. "The courts have held that clean, intermittent catheterization is necessary to help the child benefit from and have access to special education and related services." (National Dissemination Center for Children with Disabilities, retrieved September 16, 2006, from http://www.nichcy.org/pubs/fact she/fs12txt.htm, p. 2). Professionals and parents will have to design a successful bladder management program that is incorporated into the child's school day. Many children will learn to catheterize themselves during the elementary school years.

The level of the spinal cord lesion determines the child's capacity for movement as well as the need for orthotics and other assisted devices. Splinting and bracing must begin during infancy to develop appropriate upright posture and limb positioning. Preambulatory devices assist children with standing and walking at approximately the same age as peers. Standing benefits children by improving blood circulation and other organ functioning. By the age of 2 or 3 years, children should be practicing skills for crutch-walking, even though it may later be determined that a wheelchair is the most efficient means for movement. Standing and ambulation facilitate socialization among children and permit them to engage more easily in unstructured peer play and organized movement programs.

Early intervention in all developmental domains help children prepare for future school years. Ongoing therapy, medical care and/or surgical treatments are needed to manage complications throughout the individual's life. Treatment of spina bifida is best managed by a multidisciplinary team including parents, educational and medical professionals. Due to paralysis causing an imbalance between muscle

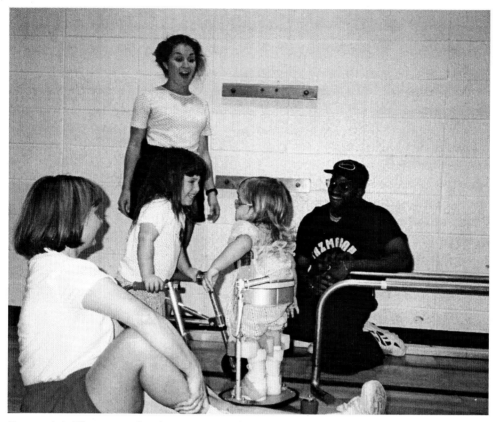

Figure 4.4. These preschoolers with spina bifida demonstrate different levels of movement skills and use of adaptive equipment.

groups, posture and orthopedic issues remain a concern for the movement therapist as a child grows and develops. The importance of upper body strength is critical to the life-time functioning of an individual with spina bifida and compensation must occur due to the inefficient use of the lower body (see Figure 4.4).

Beginning during infancy, emphasis should be on development of balance, head and trunk control, and upper extremity strength and coordination. Not only are strength and balance major movement goals during infancy and preschool ages, the child must adapt these elements in discovering new ways to accomplish daily, functional, play and movement patterns. Push or pull-toys, scooter-board activities, vestibular ball exercises, air mattress activities, fitness programs, free-weight training and swimming can be utilized during unstructured play or during instruction with the movement specialist.

Major goals (even at the preschool level) are to control weight and develop and maintain fitness that lead to life-time conditioning. The National Center on Physical Activity and Disability (NCPAD, 2004) recognizes the importance of strength training, weight control, wheelchair cardiovascular activities, and aerobic routines for individuals with spina bifida. Since visual motor functioning is impaired, training activities that include eye tracking, object focus, form discrimination, figure-ground perception, visual coordination and pursuit, and eye-hand coordination should become a part of the motor program. Balloon activities, blowing "bubbles," swinging ball exercises, chalkboard activities, bean bag and ball activities can be included in the motor program. During all physical activity, including unstructured play, adults and the child with spina bifida need to be highly aware of the occurrence of bruises, cuts, sprains, etc. due to the child's lack of feeling in lower limbs. Skin breakdown and temperature control are also major concerns that must be monitored by the movement specialist.

Hydrocephalus. This is a complication occurring from hemorrhage within the ventricular system, interruption of circulation, or reabsorption of cerebral spinal fluid (as in myelomenigocele) causing a back-up of fluid, increased intracranial pressure, and expansion of the ventricles. Often surgical placement of a ventriculo-peritoneal (VP) shunt is required which drains cerebral spinal fluid from the brain to the abdominal cavity preventing major developmental delays.

A child's growth rate may exceed the functioning potential of the size of his/her shunt causing the shunt to become obstructed. In this instance, the cerebral spinal fluid is prevented from properly draining into the peritoneum (the lining of the abdominal cavity). A blockage may occur at any time, including during a child's participation in an early intervention program. The child may appear to not feel well and may exhibit unusually poor feeding skills. A progressive series of observable abnormalities may occur: irritability and restlessness moving to an increased state of lethargy, projectile vomiting, seizures, and semi-consciousness with the eyes half-opened/half-closed (sunset eyes). Attempts to arouse the child may be unsuccessful. At this time, emergency procedures should be implemented.

Microcephaly. Microcephaly is an unusually small head circumference defined by decrease in size of 2 standard deviations below the mean. It is caused by numerous intrauterine insults and genetic disorders. During pregnancy microcephaly may be caused by exposure to toxic agents (e.g., drugs, alcohol, radiation, and chemicals), genetic and chromosomal abnormalities, and infections. Secondary causes of microcephaly include trauma during the birth process, decreased oxygen, and infections (Howard et al., 1997).

Prader-Willi Syndrome. Approximately 70 percent of infants affected have a partial deletion of chromosome 15 (15 at qllql3) which is mostly paternal in origin. Abnormalities include mild to moderate mental retardation, an obsession for eating, and subsequent serious obesity and hypotonia. The mother may have reported very little fetal movement and the child is usually born in the breech position. Feeding problems associated with respiratory difficulties may necessitate a gastrostomy. Due to feeding problems, hypotonia becomes more significant. Mental delays will often be assessed due to lack of developmental performance.

In addition, behavior problems are prevalent and often associated with ingenious "acting out" methods of attaining food. The onset of obesity occurs early from 6 months to 6 years. Gross motor exercise programs should be established. Early intervention programs should emphasize the establishment of principles for dietary habits of the child and family and caloric intake must be greatly restricted. Risk of recurrence is extremely rare (Howard et al., 1997; Kurtz et al., 1996; Widerstrom et al., 1991).

Congenital Infections

Infections may be passed through the mother's placenta and infect the fetus, resulting in illnesses that affect the newborn. The acronym TORCH reflects the commonly encountered diseases, toxoplasmosis, rubella, cytomegalovirus, herpes, and syphilis, which cause some similar malformations in the fetus. Other viruses, human immunodeficiency virus (HIV) and hepatitis B are rapidly increasing, while other infections, such as bacterial meningitis continue to remain prevalent.

Toxoplasmosis

Toxoplasmosis results from a parasite, toxoplasma protozoan, which is transmitted from the mother to the fetus. Although it is a rare cause of birth defects, 40–50 percent of children born to mothers with the parasite will be affected. The mother often contracts the infection through ingesting uncooked meat or through contact with the parasite in cat litter boxes or flower gardens; however, the protozoan is also found in some birds and reptiles. Although the mother typically is asymptomatic, the developing fetus may be severely affected if the infection occurs during the first trimester of development. Damage to the fetus can often be detected in cerebral calcifications through ultrasound. Infants may have microcephaly, deafness, retinitis, blindness, jaundice, seizures, large lymph nodes, pneumonia, and enlarged liver and spleen (Lee, 1988). However, if the disease is contracted during the third trimester, the child may be minimally affected. Some children show no symptoms until after the first year of life. Drug treatment is available for the mother with toxoplasmosis, but most drugs are not effective for treating an infected infant.

Rubella

Rubella (German measles) contracted by the mother during the first four months of pregnancy may result in abnormal physical anomalies or developmental disabilities in the newborn. Although the disease symptoms in the mother are slight (e.g., rash, low grade fever), the effects on the fetus are variable. Some effects may be transient while others are permanent. Some effects are evidenced at birth while other postnatal effects are subtle and appear over time. The most common persistent problems are hearing loss, visual problems (e.g., cataracts and glaucoma), heart disease, and mental retardation. Other symptoms include low birth weight, large liver and spleen, bone development abnormalities, meningitis, behavioral and language disorders, hernias and undescended testes. The licensing of the rubella vaccine in the 1970s has limited the number of infected children; however, there is not any specific treatment of the disease in newborns (Howard et al., 1997).

Cytomegalovirus (CMV)

Cytomegalovirus is a herpes virus that may be passed across the placenta in utero or contracted as the newborn ascends through the birth canal. It is the most common viral cause of brain damage, mental retardation, and hearing loss in unborn children. The infection occurs in 1–2 percent of live births (60–80% adults are positive for CMV). As with other herpes viruses, the infected mother may have no obvious symptoms, but during decreased resistance, the organisms may become activated. The mother may have flu-like symptoms during pregnancy that indicate the virus. If maternal illness occurs during the first trimester, fetal anomalies such as microcephaly, mental retardation, neurological defects (cerebral palsy), blindness or deafness may result. Other neonatal symptoms of infection include enlarged spleen, jaundice, petechiae (bleeding spots), microcephaly, prematurity, and chorioretinitis (Boppana, Fowler, Vaid, Hedlund, Stagno, Britt, & Pass, 1997; Howard et al., 1997; Peterson, 1987; Stagno & Whitley, 1985; Tarr, Haas, & Christie, 1996). Later maternal infection produces more subtle physical indicators in the newborn such as hearing loss or inner ear infection (Hanshaw, Dudgeon, & Marshall, 1985). At present, there is not a maternal immunization available to counteract this widespread virus nor is there specific treatment for the child virus.

Herpes

Herpes type 1 and type 2 may affect the fetus or newborn. Type 1 is predominantly an oral organism that manifests as cold sores and fever blisters, while type 2 is primarily a genital organism. Herpes is an aggressive virus that may appear in the newborn as a localized infection, but may spread to a systemic disease. Even if mothers are asymptomatic at time of delivery, the newborn may become infected. Antiviral treatment of the localized infection often prevents the spread of the disease to a generalized illness; however, treatment of a generalized illness often results in serious effects. Lethargy, respiratory distress, temperature instability, enlarged liver and spleen, poor blood coagulation, and jaundice are common symptoms in the newborn (Corey & Spear, 1986a, 1986b). Growth delay, skin scarring, retinal lesions, and microcephaly may also occur (Batshaw, 2002).

Syphilis

This disease is caused by a microorganism, Treponema palladium, that is passed from mother to newborn through the placenta, or as the baby moves through the birth canal. The severity of the disease depends on the baby's response to the infections which may invade any organ of the body. Nervous and circulatory system development may be affected. Attributes of congenital syphilis include dry skin rash, bruising, hypotonia, anemia, large liver and spleen, jaundice (Narbarro, 1954), heart defects, cataracts, deafness, and bone deformities (Peterson, 1987). However, the illness may not be detected until the child is several months old, whereby symptoms include joint swelling, limited movement or paralysis of the extremities, blindness, and hydrocephaly. Syphilis is treated with penicillin or other antibiotics and long-term disabilities may be minimal.

Human Immunodeficiency Virus (HIV)

HIV is a virus that manifests itself as an infection and may result in a disease termed Acquired Immune Deficiency Syndrome (AIDS). Individuals who are infected with HIV are referred to as HIV positive. HIV is transmitted from mother to infant through the placenta during delivery, by breast feeding or by intimate contact with body secretions (Cowan, Hellman & Chudwin, 1984; Gonik & Hammill, 1990; Howard et al., 1997). An infant may test positive for infection for up to 18 months due to maternally transferred antibodies; however, two-thirds to three-quarters of infants are not infected (Kuntz, 1996). For children that continue to test HIV positive, "On average, children progress to moderate symptoms in the second year of life and then remain moderately symptomatic for more than half of their expected lives, underscoring their need for clinical care before the onset of AIDS" (Barnhart, Caldwell, Thomas, Mascola, Ortiz, Hsu, Schulte, Parrott, Maldonado, Byers & the Pediatric Spectrum of Disease Clinical Consortium, 1996, p. 710). If an infant is without serious AIDS-defining clinical conditions during the first 2-year period, the child will probably also be free from neurological problems during this time period (Belman, Muenz, Marcus, Goedert, Landesman, Rubinstein, Goodwin, Durako, & Willoughby, 1996).

The most common features for neonates with HIV infection that progresses to AIDS include: failure-to-thrive, enlarged lymph nodes, liver, spleen, and heart, respiratory infections and pneumonia, and fevers. Pneumonia is the most prevalent problem associated with survival of neonates. However, many infected neonates appear relatively healthy without any of these symptoms present at birth.

Caretakers and professionals continue to be concerned about the spread of HIV, although transmission is much more difficult than was previously considered. For the spread of the virus to occur, the virus must be in a potentially infectious body fluid (e.g., blood, semen, vaginal secretions), it must have a route of entry to the uninfected person (e.g., break in the skin, eyes, nose, rectum, vagina), and it must be present in sufficient quantity (either large volume or repeated exposure). Caregivers should assess their level of risk in any situation and utilize universal precautions for infection control (Howard et al., 1997; Mok, Giaquinto, & DeRossi, 1987). Infection control procedures are summarized in Table 4.1.

Hepatitis B Virus (HBV)

HBV has increased in the United States due to immigration from underdeveloped countries such as Africa and Southeast Asia. When a pregnant woman is infected with HBV, the neonate has a 50 percent chance of acquiring the infection. Once born, the baby can receive protective immunoglobulins to prevent serious debilitation. Effects of the virus can produce severe systemic illness with jaundice, fever, and rash. HBV immunization of all infants is recommended by the American Academy of Pediatrics (Kurtz et al., 1996).

HBV can be transmitted to other individuals through body secretions such as saliva, wound excretions, blood, semen, vaginal secretions, and breast milk. However, it is important to note that saliva does not pose a high risk for transmission unless it is contaminated with blood. Universal precautions for infection control should be undertaken by all professionals and caretakers.

Table 4.1. Universal Infection Control Procedures.

Strict avoidance of contact with body fluids.

Wear Latex gloves during any time of possible contact with body fluids, e.g. when wiping nose or drool, administering first aid, during diaper change (change gloves after removing dirty diaper and prior to putting on new diaper).

To remove gloves, pull them off your hands by pulling them inside out.

Cover any open sores or wounds with a band-aid.

Have a 1:10 solution of bleach and water or wet wipes covered with alcohol within your reach (but not the child's reach) at all times. Bleach provides a more immediate effect than alcohol. A new solution of bleach and water should be mixed daily.

continued

Table 4.1. Universal Infection Control Procedures–*Continued.*

Before and after each session, clean all mats, toys, diapering tables, etc. with the disinfectant.

Immediately remove mouthed toys from other children's access.

Frequent handwashing is the #1 prevention of the spread of germs.

Remove watch, rings, and bracelets prior to washing hands.

When: before and after work
        before and after toileting
        before and after diapering
        before preparing/serving food
        after wiping nose
        after administering first aid
        between hands-on contact with each child

How: For at least 10 seconds, vigorously rub hands with warm water and antibacterial soap, cleansing the wrist, back of hand, palms, between fingers, and under finger nails. (Sing "Happy Birthday" twice to determine length of washing time.)

Turn off faucet and open restroom door with paper towel in clean hand to prevent recontaminating hands by touching dirty faucet and door handle; activate air dryer with back of wrist or elbow.

Sensory Impairments

Visual Impairments

Visual Impairments (after correction) which may significantly interfere with normal development in various domains include amblyopia, strabismus, and retinopathy of prematurity (see Figure 4.5).

Amblyopia refers to problems with the eye's fusional reflexes that interfere with focusing of one eye (lazy eye).

Strabismus refers to eye muscles that are not in balance causing a problem with visual alignment of the eyes (crossed-eyes).

Retinopathy of prematurity is a disorder that interrupts the vascularization of the maturing retina. It is caused by low birth weight, gestation age, and oxygen therapy (too much oxygen).

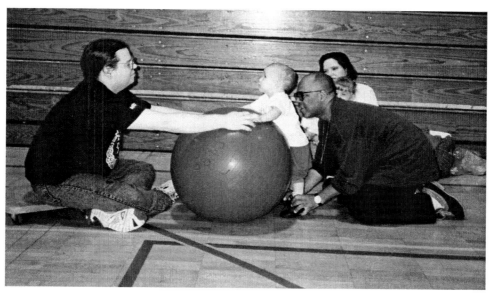

Figure 4.5. Activities for children with visual impairments must be taught through other sensory modalities. This infant is receiving active guidance, tactile discrimination, and vestibular stimulation.

Auditory Impairments

Auditory impairments, either permanent or fluctuating, may significantly interfere with normal development. Infants that are at high risk for hearing impairments include those with:

Congenital TORCH infections
Birth weight less than 1,500 grams
Hyperbilirubinemia
Perinatal asphyxia
Bacterial meningitis

Orthopedic and Neurologic Conditions

Cerebral Palsy

Cerebral palsy is a nonprogressive neuromuscular condition resulting from damage to the central nervous system during the early stages of development. Cerebral palsy results from prenatal causes in 30 percent of the cases, as a result of the birth process in 60 percent of the cases, or as a result of complications or problems after birth in 10 percent of the cases (Dunn & Leitschuh, 2006). It affects muscle tone, movement, reflexes, and posture. Although damage to the brain is not progressive in nature, deformities may increase throughout an individual's life. Anatomical features and etiologies of individuals with cerebral palsy are diverse; however, the individual's intentions for movement do not correspond with subsequent motor responses (see Figure 4.6). Cerebral palsy can be categorized according to the site of damage to the central nervous system (see Chapter 2), the extent of the brain damage (mild, moderate, severe), and the parts of the body affected (e.g., hemiplegia, triplegia, diplegia, quadriplegia) (Sherrill, 2004).

The types of cerebral palsy are generally classified according to the muscle tone abnormality or type of muscle movements that are evidenced (Dunn & Leitschuh, 2006; Howard et al., 1997; Levitt, 1982;

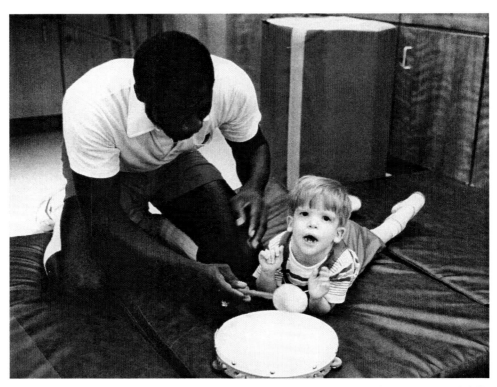

Figure 4.6. Abnormal muscle tone and reflex activity interfere with this young child's ability to progress through developmental motor milestones.

Scherzer & Tscharnuter, 1990; Sherrill, 2004). The four major types include:

Spastic Cerebral Palsy. Spastic cerebral palsy is the most common type, and is a result from damage to the pyramidal tract of the brain. In addition, there is increased motor neuronal excitability and enhanced stretch-evoked synaptic excitation of motor neurons (Van Deusen & Brunt, 1997). Muscle tightening and muscle resistance to movement, as well as a "jack knife" response (initial hyperresistance to movement at the joint followed by a sudden release) are evidenced. Hypertonia (high muscle tone) limits joint movement and contributes to the development of deformities in the spine and limbs.

Athetoid Cerebral Palsy. Athetoid cerebral palsy or dyskinesia is characterized by slow, writhing, excessive movements that are accentuated during voluntary movement attempts. Fluctuations in muscle tone as well as coordination of posture, tone and locomotion of an individual are affected due to damage to the extrapyramidal tract of the brain. Facial muscles are more often affected with this type of cerebral palsy, thus a young child may experience problems sucking, swallowing, drooling, and speaking. Stability needed for sitting and walking is also affected due to variations in muscle tone.

Ataxic cerebral palsy. Ataxic cerebral palsy affects a child's ability to coordinate hand movements and to balance during walking. It results from damage to the cerebellum. A child typically exhibits uncoordinated movements and an awkward gait. Due to exaggerated movements in attempts to balance and continued efforts to stabilize, rigid movements may result.

The term **mixed cerebral palsy** is applied to individuals when more than one type of cerebral palsy is prevalent but one type is not dominant. Significant motor control problems are apparent due to tenseness of movement (spastic) and lack of movement control (athetosis) (Dunn & Leitschuh, 2006). Due to central nervous system damage, movement disorders are frequently accompanied by disorders of other systems. Intellectual deficits, hearing and vision problems, seizure disorders (Thurman & Widerstrom, 1990), and growth retardation (Thommessen, Kase, Riis, & Heiberg, 1991) are often evidenced. Additionally, as a result of motor difficulties, self-help skills (e.g., dressing) are limited. Feeding problems are exhibited by approximately 48 percent of individuals with cerebral palsy, and correspondingly, nutritional status and energy levels are compromised

(Thommessen et al., 1991).

Two other types of cerebral palsy may infrequently be found in evaluations of children with cerebral palsy: **rigid cerebral palsy** and **tremor cerebral palsy**. Rigid cerebral palsy is very severe. It is the result of damage to the extrapyramidal tract and is characterized by severely limited movement due to hypertensity of flexor and extensor muscles. Hyperextension of body parts, postural defects and severe mental retardation are often present. Tremor cerebral palsy results from damage to the cerebellum or basal ganglia and may result in uncontrolled involuntary and rhythmic movements which may either be present at all times or only during movement attempts.

Seizures

Seizures result from an electric-chemical imbalance in the regulatory center of the brain (Dunn & Leitschuh, 2006), and the condition of epilepsy results when seizures are recurrent (Howard et al., 1997). All humans have a threshold for seizures, but the threshold is not typically reached. It is presumed that each individual's threshold is genetically determined and interactive with environmental events (Brunquell, 1994). The risk of seizures increases with conditions such as perinatal trauma, fetal distress, congenital and postnatal infection, drugs, tumors, and chromosomal abnormalities.

The International Classification of Epileptic Seizures categorized seizures as **partial** (begins in a portion of one cerebral hemisphere) or **generalized** (involves both cerebral hemispheres) (Batshaw, 2002; Howard et al., 1997). Generalized seizures can be further categorized as **absence (petit mal)**, **tonic-clonic (grand-mal)**, **myoclonic**, and **atonic**. Partial seizures are classified as **simple partial or complex partial seizures**.

An **absence** seizure involves unconsciousness for approximately 1–15 seconds, suspending mental processes and physical activity. Muscle twitching and eye rolling or blinking may occur frequently throughout the day and may be the only observable signs of a seizure.

A **tonic-clonic** seizure includes a tonic, a clonic, and a sleep phase. During the tonic phase, the body stiffens in rigid muscular contraction and consciousness is lost. During the clonic phase, jerking, uncontrolled body movements occur, and respiration and swallowing is interrupted. Sleep generally follows these two phases. General confusion and headache symptoms may also follow a seizure. Tonic clonic seizures resulting from a young child having a high temperature are termed **febrile seizures**. Other frequent causes of tonic-clonic seizures are inborn errors of metabolism (i.e., congenital enzyme deficiency such as PKU), traumatic brain injury, and meningitis (Batshaw, 2002; Howard et al., 1997).

Myoclonic seizures are brief, sudden violent contractions that may occur in one body part or in the entire body. Infantile spasms are a classic example of myoclonic seizures. Most often occurring between the ages of 6 months to 24 months, the child will exhibit neurological and mental regression. Disabilities that may be associated with infantile spasms include Down syndrome, tuberous sclerosis, congenital infections, birth asphyxia, and PKU.

Atonic seizures are characterized by sudden and momentary loss of muscle tone whereby the child may sag or collapse. The child may also lose consciousness. Thus, atonic seizures have the opposite appearance of myoclonic seizures.

The two types of seizures classified as partial seizures are simple partial seizures (previously known as Jacksonian seizures) and complex partial seizures (previously known as psychomotor seizures or temporal lobe seizures). During simple partial seizures consciousness is not lost, while during partial seizures, consciousness is lost (Batshaw, 2002; Howard et al., 1997).

Simple partial seizures may be exemplified in various forms. An *aura* may occur from the frontal, parietal, temporal, or occipital lobes resulting in different behaviors. If the seizure originates in the temporal lobe, the child may experience psychic symptoms associated with smell, sound, and taste or emotional experiences such as fear, anger, or laughter. If the seizure originates in the occipital or parietal lobes, visual hallucinations may occur. A *focal-motor seizure* results in muscular twitching which begins in one area of the body and may spread to the entire body. Another type of simple partial seizure occurs with *autonomic symptoms* involving the involuntary functions controlled by the brain. During the onset of this type of seizure, the child may experience increased heart rate, discoloring of the face, and discomfort in the chest or abdomen. These behaviors should not be confused with breathholding spells, which may have similar symptoms.

Complex partial seizures are most common in older children, but may occur during infancy. Although these seizures resemble generalized absence seizures, they are preceded by an aura, last longer than 10 seconds, and the child is either confused or sleeps following the seizure. The actual seizure often involves repetitive motor movements, i.e., lip smacking, groaning, chewing, and eye blinking. These seizures are frequently controlled with medication (Batshaw, 2002).

The effects of seizures on cognitive functioning are associated with type, age of onset, and frequency. In general, an earlier onset leads to a poorer prognosis. Each seizure has the potential for causing brain injury due to lessening of neurological metabolites. Generally, diminished concentration and mental processing result from continuous seizures in children (Howard et al., 1997).

Procedures for management of a seizure include the following: protect the child from falling and hitting her head, do not try to prevent the child from having a seizure or physically restrain her during a seizure, try to lay the child on her side and provide support under her head to prevent choking or aspiration and loosen the child's clothing. DO NOT put anything in her mouth. If the seizure lasts 10–15 minutes or there is a continuous repetition of seizures, emergency medical procedures should be implemented (i.e., call for an ambulance). Following the seizure activity, the child should be allowed to rest or sleep as needed.

Hypoxia Ischemic Encephalopathy

This neurological condition occurs immediately following birth and is a result of severe asphyxiation. Placenta previa, abrupto placenta, prolapsed cord, cephalopelvic disproportion and prolonged labor are causes of asphyxia. Damage to the brain from asphyxiation occurs due to lack of oxygen (hypoxia), lack of circulation (ischemia) and acidosis. The site of the damage to the brain and the severity of asphyxiation determine the resulting disorders. Subtle damage may result in attention-deficit-hyperactivity disorder (ADHD) or learning disabilities, while more severe damage may result in quadriplegia cerebral palsy, mental retardation and seizures. Damage to the brain and specific abnormality patterns can be visualized with ultrasound, computed tomography (CT scan), or magnetic resonance imaging (MRI) (Batshaw, 2002).

Significant Intracranial Hemorrhage

Intraventricular Hemorrhage (IVH) (Grade III or IV)

IVH is an extremely serious and common neurological disorder of premature infants. Grades or levels are characterized by hemorrhage or bleeding and the areas of the brain tissue that are effected. Levels I and II include bleeding which is isolated to the subependymal germinal matrix and contained to normal ventricle size. Levels III and IV have indications of severe bleeding with acute ventricular dilation and increased pressure and hemorrhage into tissues of the cerebral cortex. IVH is usually diagnosed by ultrasound or CAT scan (Brann, 1985; Papille, Munsick-Bruno, & Schaefer, 1983).

Periventricular Leukomalcia (PVL)

Due to premature birth, PVL leads to hemorrhage in the ventricles of the brain. These areas of brain tissue control movements of the lower limbs, thus hemorrhage may cause spastic diplegia (the more common type of cerebral palsy associated with prematurity). Hemorrhage (intracranial bleeding) may occur prenatally or postnatally and is often associated with birth asphyxia. Infants will have a very poor neurodevelopmental outcome (Batshaw, 2002; Clark, Dykes, Bachman & Ashurst, 1996).

Technology Dependence

With the advances in technology many infants with serious medical conditions are surviving; however, the incidence of developmental delay may increase due to procedures such as home oxygen, home ventilation, tracheostomy, and gastrostomy feeding (see Figure 4.7). Many young children are receiving early intervention services while utilizing these technologies. It is therefore important for service providers to understand the care and contraindications associated with their use.

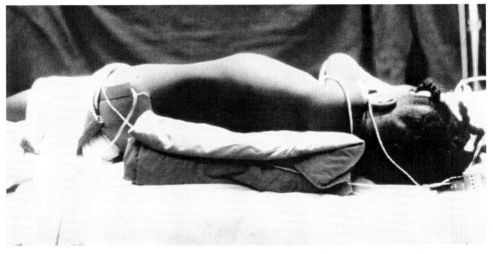

Figure 4.7. NICU provides several "life cords" for this child as he recovers from trauma.

Respiratory Distress Syndrome (RDS)

RDS occurs in preterm infants. It is caused by the absence of necessary surfactant which prevents the lungs from collapsing during normal breathing (Batshaw, 2002; Enhorning, Shennan, & Possmayer, 1985). Infants with RDS often spend a substantial period of time in a Neonatal Intensive Care Unit (NICU) and may have additional delays caused by this experience. Treatment for RDS includes maintaining a continuous positive airway pressure to keep the alveoli (air pockets of the lungs) open and providing adequate exchange of oxygen and carbon dioxide. Ventilators are often needed for this process.

Bronchopulmonary Dysplasia (BPD)

BPD is a chronic lung disease caused by respiratory distress soon after birth requiring mechanical ventilation and supplemental oxygen. Most children can be slowly removed or weaned off ventilator assistance in several weeks. Trauma associated with high inflation pressures, **barotrauma**, may be a cause of BPD. In addition, other causes of BPD include infection, asphyxia, and meconium aspiration (inhalation of feces into lung passages with first respiratory efforts). Abnormal tissue changes occur resulting in pulmonary function abnormalities including decreased pulmonary compliance, abnormal lung volumes, and airway resistance. As a result, the infant must increase exerted efforts or work harder to breathe comfortably. The child may be dependent on oxygen therapy and diuretics to decrease airway resistance (Able-Boone, 1993; Batshaw, 1993; Kugelman, Durand, & Garg, 1997; Louch, 1993).

Tracheostomy

Infants who have experienced severe respiratory trauma during or after the birth process may need a tracheostomy. A tracheostomy is an opening in the trachea (windpipe) that the infant will breathe through instead of the nose and mouth. A short piece of plastic is surgically placed in the hole in the windpipe and does not connect to the lungs. The tracheostomy is not permanent and can be removed after problems have been corrected or when the child grows and may no longer need the tracheostomy. Caregivers will not be able to hear the infant cry or talk at first, but eventually the child can learn to communicate. At first the baby will have a home apnea alarm (monitor) to indicate if the infant is not breathing or if the heart beat is too slow (bradycardia) (Batshaw, 2002; Church & Glennen, 1992).

Problems that may affect the infant's respiratory system include many different birth defects or disabililties. Often an infant is premature and the lungs are not fully developed. The lungs do not possess the necessary surfactant (lubricant) to facilitate adequate lung expansion. The infant must be placed in NICU and on a ventilator and oxygen therapy. Oxygen therapy may result in additional long-term problems causing ventilator dependency. A child's dependency on mechanical ventilation is directly related to the problems that caused respiratory failure. Children on ventilators are also more likely to have nutritional problems due to gastroesophageal reflux, vomiting, oral motor dysfunctions, and acute illness (Enhorning et al., 1985; Kettrick & Donar, 1985; Sindel, Maisels & Ballantine, 1989; Starrett, 1991).

Several processes need to be understood regarding cleaning and maintenance of the tracheostomy (Lichtenstein, 1986; Kennelly, 1990). Feeding is performed as with a typical baby. If a young child has a tracheostomy, the teacher should be informed by the caregiver or medical professional of any necessary procedures. Often the teacher must ask questions of the family. The information that a professional should be aware of in order to be properly informed include: (a) changing the ties holding the tube in place, (b) cleaning the opening (stoma) of the tracheostomy, (c) changing the tracheostomy tube, and (d) emergency procedures to use if breathing should stop and cardiopulmonary resuscitation (CPR) must be started.

Changing the ties holding tube in place. The ties holding the tube in place should be changed daily by the family or caregiver. However, if the ties become loose, wet, dirty, or the knot of the ties is pressing too hard against the baby's skin, it may be necessary for the teacher to change the ties while the child is attending child care or school. **Do not change the tracheostomy ties by yourself unless absolutely necessary**. One person should assist holding the infant in place while the other individual replaces the ties. These steps should be followed: (a) suction the tube to decrease chances of coughing up mucus; (b) place a towel roll under shoulders of infant to better expose the tracheostomy area; c) insert new ties under old ties and then remove old ties; and (d) while ties are loosened, examine child's neck for redness, rash, or irritation. Ties should be replaced so that one finger can easily be slipped under the tie.

Cleaning the tracheostomy opening (stoma) may be necessary, especially when a strong odor is present. The area around the stoma should be carefully cleaned using a Q-tip dipped in half-strength hydrogen peroxide and rinsed with a Q-tip dipped in water. The tracheostomy tube should be held in place with a finger while cleaning around the stoma. Dry the area with a 4x4 inch gauze pad. **Do not use powders or lotions on the skin around the stoma**. If a skin irritation or rash is present, the caregiver should be advised to obtain the necessary ointments from the physician.

Changing the tracheostomy tube is not a routine procedure for which the early intervention professional should be responsible for perfoming. However, the professional should know the procedures in case of emergency. The tracheostomy tube should be suctioned before starting the procedure. Attach ties to a new or clean tube. A cover or obturator should be inserted in the new tube opening to serve as a guide for easy insertion. A blanket roll should be placed under the infant's neck. The infant should be restrained so to prevent excess movement during the procedure. Cut the old ties and remove the old tube (see Figure 4.8).

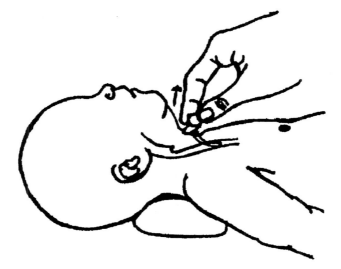

Figure 4.8. Remove old tube while a partner stabilizes the child.

Using one hand lift the tube using an up-and-out motion (see Figure 4.9).

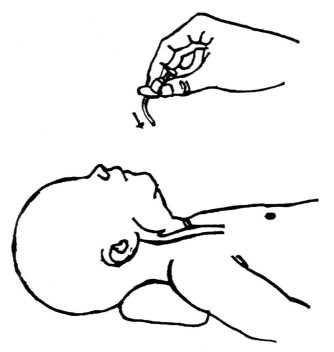

Figure 4.9. Insert a new tube by using an "in and downward" motion.

Insert the new tube gently and remove the obturator as soon as the tube is in place. The child cannot breathe until the obturator is removed from the opening (see Figure 4.10).

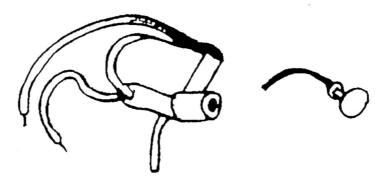

Figure 4.10. Remove obturator from tube immediately after inserting tube.

Tie the tracheostomy tube in place as described in previous section. The infant may cough, cry, turn red, and sweat during the process. Always talk to the infant during the process using a calming tone of voice.

Signs of breathing problems may include restlessness, increased respiratory rate, heavy or labored breathing, noisy breathing, retractions of breastbone and skin between the ribs, blue or pale color, sweating, or a whistling noise coming from the tracheostomy tube. **Bleeding** from the tube should be reported to caregiver and reported to a physician immediately.

CPR with a **tracheostomy** should be performed if the infant stops breathing. Make sure the tube ties are tied. **Suction the tracheostomy tube at once**. If the tube is blocked with mucus and the baby is still not breathing after suction, call for help and begin CPR. If the tube has come out, replace it as described in the previous section. After tube is replaced and the baby is still not breathing, call for help and begin CPR. Place your mouth or an ambu bag over the tube opening to form a seal when performing CPR (see Figure 4.11).

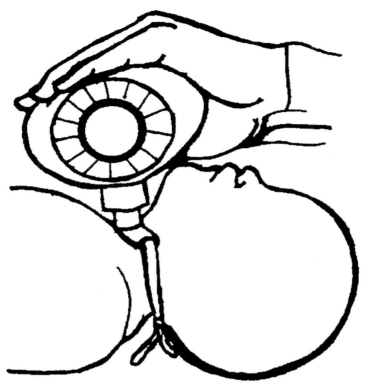

Figure 4.11. To perform CPR with a tracheostomy, place your mouth or attach an ambu bag over tube to form seal.

Each early intervention program should have established emergency and treatment procedures. If the early intervention professional is being required to perform procedures routinely that should be done by the family or caregiver, a conference should be arranged with the intervention team that is providing qualified services to the infant. However, the professional should be prepared to handle emergencies for plugged tracheostomy tubes, occasional coughing out of the tube, vomiting, and feeding.

Gastrostomy

A gastrostomy is performed surgically when infants are not able to suck or swallow enough nutrients for adequate and proper oral nutrition. A tube is placed directly into the stomach of the baby for feeding and is kept in place by a special dressing. Conditions which may lead to the need for a gastrostomy include structural problems with the tongue or mouth (cleft palate), weak oral-motor musculature, hyperactive gag reflex, short-gut syndrome, neurological problems, and ventilator assistance (Batshaw, 2002; Howard et al., 1997; Luiselli & Luiselli, 1995; Sontag, 1990).

To assist the early interventionist, caregivers should provide the child's medical instructions. Cleaning and care of the gastrostomy tube and cleansing of the stoma is a "must" and should be done at home.

During feeding, a liquid formula or processed foods from a blender are administered in small amounts (i.e., 2–3 cc's/minute finishing in about 20 minutes). A large syringe should be used to feed the child and also to administer medications. Feeding should flow by gravity and occur slowly. The syringe should be held above the child, but should never be left suspended and unattended. After feeding, the baby should be placed on the right side or on the stomach with the body propped at a 30 degree angle.

The doctor should be called if bloody residuals are noticed, if the stomach seems enlarged and the baby is uncomfortable for over an hour, if the tube cannot be replaced, if a tissue build-up begins to develop around the stoma, or if there is a consistent, unpleasant smell coming from the stoma.

The early intervention professional should be familiar with the gastrostomy tube. If the tube should come out, the opening (stoma) may close within 3 hours; therefore, the child's caregiver should be called immediately to replace the tube. In the event the tube must be replaced while under the care of the early interventionist, the following procedures should be implemented: (a) place tip of clean tube into the opening or the stoma; (b) push the tube until about 1 inch beyond the bulb; (c) fill the bulb with 5 cc's of tap water; (d) gently pull the bulb into position against the stomach wall; (e) secure the outside portion of the tube by using a stoma adhesive dressing and tape in place.

Gastroschisis

Gastroschisis is a congenital defect of the abdominal wall and typically appears to be to the right of the umbilical cord. It has no sac and commonly is in the area of the midgut and stomach. The intestine is thickened, shortened, and usually malrotated. The best description is given by Turnell (1993) as, "failure of vascularization of the abdominal wall, likely secondary to complete dissolution of the right umbilical vein at a time before collateral circulation can maintain integrity of the mesenchyme" (p. 547). The bowel is extruded and may include the stomach. Incidence is approximately one in 4,000 live births.

By 13 weeks gestation, gastroschisis can be diagnosed allowing for prompt preparation for repair of infants with this abdominal wall defect. The infant will suffer health-based delays due to needing surgical repair; however, if these procedures are not performed early, the child will have a greatly oversized abdominal cavity and large protruding stomach. With prenatal diagnosis and immediate surgical repair there is high survival rate, good prognosis and minimal complications. Mechanical ventilation will be necessary, but should be discontinued in 48–72 hours. Children with other coexisting congenital anomalies may need further consideration during the postoperative period.

Exposure to Known Teratogens or Drugs

Fetal Alcohol Syndrome (FAS)

Fetal alcohol syndrome (FAS) was first reported by Lemoine of Nantes, France, in 1968; however, his report was not well accepted. His study described the multiple effect of alcohol on the fetus and was rediscovered in 1973 by Jones and Smith (Jones, 1997).

> Basic scientific research on embryonic and fetal development has confirmed that alcohol is teratogenic. Epidemiologic studies have shown it to be the most prevalent human teratogen to which humans are exposed. Unlike many teratogenic exposure in humans, alcohol use can vary considerably in both the timing of exposure and the amount of consumption across the gestational period, with alcoholic mothers having the most frequent and highest consumption. (Swayze, Johnson, Hanson, Piven, Sato, Giedd, Mosnik, & Andreasen, 1997)

"FAS is considered to be the most common environmental cause of mental retardation in the developed countries" (Stromland & Hellstrom, 1996, p. 845). Children also may be at greater risk for developmental delay. Unfortunately, due to legal issues, it is hard to provide evidence of the true relationship of alcohol consumption and the link to mental retardation. Since mental retardation is usually defined as an IQ less than 70 and the average IQ of FAS is approximately 65, 50 percent of the population with delays may only have learning disabilities or behavioral problems which may be termed fetal alcohol effects (FAE). Abnormalities of FAS and FAE include: CNS involvement, mental retardation, learning disabilities, hyperactivity, poor physical growth, facial dysmorphism, microcephaly, short palpebral fissures (eye slits) causing eyes to appear to be wide-set, strabismus, ptosis of the eyelid, poorly formed nasal philtrum, thin upper lip, and flat maxilla. Newborns may experience severe tremors and exhibit physiological indicators which are confused with a "failure-to-thrive" interpretation (Jones, 1997; Swayze et al., 1997).

Hand development is often affected with abnormalities including small nails, mild syndactyly, and short fourth and fifth metacarpals. The hand will also show a mildly altered upper palmar crease patterning. In addition, the child will exhibit fine motor dysfunction manifested by weak grasp, poor eye-hand coordination, tremors, and hyperactivity in childhood. Infants appear to be very irritable, then demonstrate hyperactivity as children, and become very social as teenagers. The pleasant social behaviors of the adolescent lead to probable continuation of another generation of children with similar problems (Jones, 1997; Swayze et al., 1997).

The risk of FAS varies, but *does* increase with the amount of alcohol exposure (Bailey & Wolery, 1992; Coles, Smith, Fernhoff & Falek, 1985; Jones, 1997). The amount of alcohol consumed during pregnancy is considered to affect the severity of FAS. The least significant effect has been recognized as two drinks per day which causes slightly lower birth weight. When the amount was known to be four to six drinks per day, then additional clinical features become more evident. The most serious problem or consequence of heavy prenatal exposure to alcohol (eight to ten drinks per day) is brain development and function. *According to Jones (1997), ethanol or its by-products has become a major public health concern as a teratogen.*

Fetal Hydantoin Sydrome

Research data since 1968 on Fetal Hydantoin Syndrome, also known as Fetal Dilantin Sydrome, have suggested the possible teratogenic effects of anticonvulsant drugs (Fredrick, 1973; Jones, 1997; Meadow, 1968). Varying patterns of abnormalities include mild to moderate growth deficiency, borderline mental retardation, broad and depressed nasal bridge, short nose with bowed upper lip, cleft lip and palate, strabismus, hand deformities including occasional finger-like thumb, dislocation of hip, short neck, widely-spaced small nipples, low-set hairline with very coarse scalp hair, and abnormal palm crease.

Fetal Hydantoin Syndrome causes multiple effects on mental capacities with an average IQ of 71. Infants have "failure to thrive" symptoms for no particular reason. In addition to Dilantin, other anticonvulsant drugs which may cause similar problems if exposed to the fetus prenatally include carbamazepine, valproic acid, mysoline, and phenobarbital. Exposure to a combination of anticonvulsant drugs increases the risk of abnormalities of the fetus. The risk of having some effects of exposure to anticonvulsant drugs is about 33 percent.

Prenatal Exposure to Cocaine/Crack and Tobacco

Fetuses prenatally exposed to cocaine or crack have experienced the same "highs" and associated side effects as the mother. The drugs cross into the fetus through the placenta and remain in the fetal system for over four times as long as in the mother's bloodstream. Research findings (Covington, Nordstrom-Klee, Ager, Sokol, & Delaney-Black, 2002; Handler, Mason, Rosenberg, & Davis, 1994; Medline Plus, 2005; Miller-Loncar, Lester, Seifer, Lagasse, Bauer, & Shankaran, 2005; Scafidi, Field, Wheeden, Schanberg, Kuhn, Symanski, Zimmerman, & Bandstra, 1996; Shankaran, Das, Bauer, Bada, Lester, & Wright, 2004) indicated a negative impact from these substances on pre and postnatal child development. Studies reported that intrauterine growth retardation occurs from exposure to crack, cocaine, or alcohol. Newborns will go through a type of "withdrawal" which includes the following: a high pitched moaning/crying sound, hypertonicity, tremulousness, and a hypersensitivity to sensory stimuli. Infants are often born prematurely, have low birth weight, need NICU treatment for a longer than average time period, exhibit greater incidence of periventricular-intraventricular hemorrhage, have a smaller head circumference (indicating delayed brain growth), and have neurological damage. The infant may demonstrate an inferior cluster of test criteria on the *Neonatal Behavioral Assessment Scale* (Brazelton, 1984). During the sleep wake cycles, the infant may indicate difficulty maintaining alert stages and exhibit increased levels of irritability.

Long term effects from the use of drugs are manifested through behavioral actions such as hyperactivity and strong acting-out behaviors (e.g., temper tantrums, self-destructive behaviors). Perceptual-motor difficulties, slower visuomotor speed, delayed gross motor development, poor motor performance and growth retardation are physical indicators found in young children (Miller-Loncar et.al., 2005). Deficiencies in motor skills may cause frustrations while playing with toys, or other activities involving play. Therefore, the need for early intervention is highlighted.

Tobacco use by the mother has also been found to negatively impact pre and post-natal development. Frank, Augustyn, Knight, Pell, and Zuckerman (2001) reviewed studies associated with exposure to tobacco and found increased incidence of poor early motor development. Singer, Arendt, Minnes, Farkas, Salvator, and Kirchner (2002) included a substantial number of premature infants who had prenatal substance exposure to tobacco, cocaine, and alcohol, and the results indicated adverse effects on the growth, health, development and behavior of the infants. An increased risk of delayed development at 2 years of age was also found. This study also reported that moderate use of alcohol, marijuana, and crack cocaine resulted in consistent adverse effects. In a study that considered methamphetamine-exposed newborns who were also exposed to nicotine, it was reported that these newborns had significantly lower birth weight and smaller head circumferences than infants exposed to methamphetamine alone.

Psychiatric Disturbances of Infancy

It is not the intent of this textbook to address disturbances of mental health and development disorders manifested in infancy. The National Center for Clinical Infant Programs realized the need for a more sophisticated understanding of factors that contribute to maladaptive patterns of infant mental health. Diagnostic Classification: *0–3: Diagnostic Classification of Mental Health and Developmental Disorders of Infancy and Early Childhood* (National Center for Clinical Infant Programs, 1995) provides a framework which categorizes emotional and behavioral patterns that may deviate significantly from typical development.

For numerous reasons, infants with disabilities and their caregivers experience different and complex psychosocial disorders. Traumatic stress, anxiety, mood disorders of depression, grief reaction, attachment deprivation, adjustment disorders, sleep and eating behavior disorders, and multisystem developmental and pervasive developmental disorder are examples of psychiatric disturbances of infancy. It is recognized that young children need effective early intervention before deviations become consolidated, increasing secondary problems of maladaptive behaviors. Understanding the adaptive capacities of coping provides a foundation for planning and implementing effective interventions.

Infants who have experienced emotional or stress-related trauma may benefit from a developmental motor and exercise program. Reference is made in Chapter 6 to Psychological Response to Stress (PRS), a principle of "Progressive Interactive Facilitation: Principles of Intervention." All clinical programs examining the intervention treatment plans of young children with mental health and psychiatric disturbances of infancy should consider specific exercise programs as a potential method for coping with stress.

DEVELOPMENTAL DELAY

Infants and toddlers who incur medical problems often qualify for services under IDEA due to resulting developmental delay. It is important for professionals to be knowledgeable about the previously described medical conditions. However, young children who have not been diagnosed with a physical or mental condition may also be at risk for developmental delay and therefore qualify for Part C services. The delay may occur in one or more of the following areas: cognitive development, physical development (including vision and hearing), communication development, social or emotional development, and adaptive development (self-help area).

The determination of developmental delay must be made by a multidisciplinary evaluation team. The evaluation team members include the child's family or appointed caregivers and qualified professionals from the necessary disciplines closely related to the child's suspected area of delay.

PERVASIVE DEVELOPMENTAL DISORDER

Pervasive Developmental Disorder includes the following disorders:

Autistic Disorder, Rett's Disorder, Childhood Disintegrative Disorder, Asperger's Disorder, and PDD Not Otherwise Specified (Diagnostic Statistical Manual IV, American Psychiatric Association, 1994). These disorders are communication disorders and although the criteria are similar, each has unique, distinguishing qualities. The term Autism Spectrum Disorder (ASD) is frequently found in the literature, and includes 3 of the aforementioned disorders (Autism, Asperger's Disorder, and PDD Not Otherwise Specified), as well as other less discussed disorders: semantic pragmatic communication disorder, nonverbal learning disabilities, high functioning autism, hyperlexia and some aspects of ADHD (Kutscher, Atwood, & Wolff, 2005). The reported incidence of Pervasive Developmental Disorder has increased during the past 15 years (Charman, 2002; Wing & Potter, 2002). As indicated by Chakrabarti and Fombonne (2005), the rate of autism is as high as 58.7 and 62.6 per 10,000 preschoolers while other researchers indicate a rate of 1–2 per thousand (Bryson & Smith, 1998). It has been summarized that 1 in 150 children have an autism spectrum disorder (Autism Society of America, 2006). Most recently the CDC stated, "Autism disorders are more common than previously, affecting about one in 150 8-year-olds in 14 states" (Hitti, 2007).

The distinction between autism, Asperger's syndrome and pervasive developmental disorder is difficult. It is also difficult to distinguish autism spectrum disorders from developmental delay during the first 2 years of life. However, diagnosis becomes more apparent after the age of 24 months: differences between the two groups of children were found in communication and social behaviors (e.g., smiling, responding to name, joining functional play with small toys with an adult) (Trillingsgaard, Sorensen, Nemec, & Jorgensen, 2005). During the past decade, several instruments have been developed to screen a child with suspected autism. Most are questionnaires or checklists that are completed by the parent, caregiver, or physician. The Child Behavior Checklist (CBCL) (Christiansen, Houmann, Landorph, & Skovgaard, 2006), the Checklist for Autism in Toddlers (CHAT) (Baron-Cohen, Allen, & Gillberg, 1992), the Modified CHAT (Robins, Fein, Barton, & Green, 2001), the Bayley Scales (2006) and the Early Relational Assessment (ERA) (Christiansen et al., 2006) can be used to screen and/or identify children age 0–3 years. The CHAT and CBC screening instruments have questionable validity (Williams & Brayne, 2006). Therefore, it is recommended that child development indicators, observation, school or agency report, and a profile of the child's strengths and weaknesses are utilized to determine the actual diagnosis (Jones, Cork, & Chowdhury, 2006).

Although specific diagnosis may not be easily apparent, early identification of a PDD is valuable in intervention. For the diagnosis of autism, a child must have onset of symptoms before age 3 years and the child must meet 6 of the 12 criteria listed in the DSM-IV (1994).

Autistic Spectrum Disorders

Autism Spectrum Disorder (ASD) is the more recent terminolgy for pervasive developmetal disorder and therefore these terms can be used interchangeably. According to Blaxill (2004), ASD should be considered an urgent public health concern. Dr. Leo Kanner, a child psychiatrist, published the first information that he termed "autistic disturbances of affective contact" (1943, p. 217). He believed that these children had one fundamental disturbance: "an inability to relate themselves in the ordinary way to people and situations from the beginning of life" (p. 242). This description is still appropriate and is included as a part of many definitions of autism. Autism spectrum disorders is considered one of the most devastating disorders of childhood due to its prevalence, morbidity, outcome, impact on the family, and cost to society (DiCicco-Bloom, Lord, Zwaigenbaum, Courchesne, Dager, Schmitz, Schultz, Crawley, & Young, 2006).

Autism was added as a special education exceptionality in IDEA (1990) and is described in 1997 IDEA as:

- a developmental disability significantly affecting verbal and nonverbal communication and social interaction,
- generally evident before age 3 that adversely affects a child's educational performance,
- engagement in repetitive activities and stereotyped movements,
- resistance to environmental change or changes in daily routines, and
- unusual responses to sensory experiences.

The term does not apply if a child's educational performance is adversely affected primarily because the child has a serious emotional disturbance (34 C.F. R., Sec 300.7 [b] [1]).

The mechanisms underlying autism spectrum disorders (ASD) have not truly been explained or clarified, but it appears that the causes are related to various overlapping factors. Genetic factors are currently considered as the primary cause (Folstein & Rosen-Heidley, 2001), but pre-, peri-, and neonatal complications have recently been identified as frequent in children with ASD (Hoshino, Yashima, Ishige, Tachibana, Watanabe, Kaneko, & Kumashiro, 1980; Juul-Dam, Townsend, & Courchesne, 2001). A recent study found that neonatal complications (hyperbilirubinemia, premature birth, asphyxia, use of photo therapy, and respiratory distress) were significantly greater in children with ASD than with typical children (Sugie, Sugie, Fukuda, & Ido, 2005). Authors also concluded that the interaction between neonatal complications and familial factors resulted in greater incidence of ASD.

Other theories reflect neurological differences in the etiology of autism (e.g., Gilman & Newman, 1992; Graham, 1990; Miller & Lane, 2000; Westman, 1990). The neurological basis of autism is unknown; however, it appears that autism reflects neurological immaturity (a failure of brain development) and diffuse system involvement that effects several neurological sites simultaneously. Early research (Churchland, 1986) had indicated a linear model of neurological function rather than an understanding of the interrelationship and repetitiveness of function within the brain. More recent studies indicate neurological abnormalities within the brain stem, cerebellum, medial-temporal lobe and surrounding areas, and cognitive executive functions of the brain. Neurobiological differences have been evident in the cerebellum, cerebrum, amygdala and possibly hippocampus (e.g., Carper & Courchesne, 2005; Hazlett, Poe, Gerig, Smith, Provenzale, Ross, Gilmore, & Piven, 2005; Schumann, Hamstrea, Goodlin-Jones, Lotspeich, Kwon, & Buonocore, 2004). Abnormalities in brain enlargement (size and weight) have been determined by measuring head circumference. Literature also expresses that complex neurological systems are involved, and that the interaction, hierarchical network, and dynamic processes relate to the etiology of autism. These research findings impact the treatment and intervention from a movement specialist. An integrative approach among many disciplines with a focus on the dynamics between family and child-centered teams is needed. Individualistic programming is needed due to the variations of impairment between individuals.

Major symptoms of autism are deficits in sociability, deficits in reciprocal verbal and nonverbal communication, a limited range of the child's interests and activities, and sensory dysfunction. Difficulty with motor planning (dyspraxia) is common in children with autism and PDD although it is infrequently recognized (Dejean, 2006). Although the child has problems with visual perception, the visual domain is usually superior to auditory perception. Examples of sensory dysfunction include: children may sniff their food and have an intense dislike of certain tastes or textures, or children may cover their ears and stare with fascination at some visual displays and have an outstanding rote visual or auditory memory. Qualities of children with autism within each preschool developmental domain are discussed in more detail below.

Motor

Early gross and fine motor development is consistent with developmental motor milestones; however, approximately half of children with Asperger's syndrome and 67 percent of children with average or near-average intelligence demonstrate clinically significant motor impairment (Manjiviona & Prior, 1995). Although early motor development is typical, later development is more notably affected. Common findings in young children include increased joint laxity and hypotonia, clumsiness, apraxia, and toe walking. Difficulties may also occur with more complex motor behaviors such as stacking cubes or climbing on toddler/preschool playground equipment.

Motor stereotypic behaviors include hand flapping, pacing, spinning, running in circles, twirling a string, tearing paper, drumming, and flipping light switches; while oral stereotypic behaviors include humming or incessant questioning. Low level repetitive behaviors are associated with younger infants, while more complex repetitive behaviors are associated with older preschoolers (Mooney, Gray, & Tonge, 2006). Self-injurious behavior, such as biting, head banging, and gouging may also occur in children with autism.

The inability to concentrate and intrusive stereotypic behaviors such as hand flapping, may prevent children from engaging in meaningful activity or social interaction. During self-initiated activity, some children with autism have unusually long attention spans although they are unable to focus on a joint activity with another person. A child may manipulate or line up toys without apparent awareness of what the toys represent, and due to the lack of motor planning, the child may not engage in symbolic or pretend play which is typical for preschoolers. Behavior difficulties may occur when someone directs them to change activities or if a ritual behavior is interrupted.

Cognition

Approximately thirty percent of individuals with autism have no cognitive impairment, but cognitive level is significantly associated with severity of the autistic symptoms and is more frequent in males (Fombonne, 2003). Medical research has recently found an association between autism and other rare, genetically determined medical conditions such as Fragile X syndrome (Belmonte, Allen, Beckel-Mitchener, Boulanger, Carper & Webb, 2004; Wolff, 2006) and tuberous sclerosis (Fombonne, 2003). Individuals with some chromosomal anomalies may have cognitive delay. Neuropsychological testing typically reveals an uneven cognitive profile for individuals with autism, with nonverbal skills generally superior to verbal skills, except in Asperger's syndrome, whereby the reverse pattern may exist. Children have poor insight into what others are thinking and this persists throughout life. Attention is problematic. Creativity is often limited, although a limited number of individuals with autism have surprisingly good musical, mathematical, or visual-spatial abilities.

Social

Shyness, fearfulness, anxiety, and changes in mood are evidenced by young children with autism. Although some children may be affectionate, this affection may be displayed inappropriately or on the child's terms, without the expected joy and reciprocity that typical children would display. Lack of social play is apparent as the children engage most often in repetitive and stereotypic play with little imaginative play (Kanner, 1943) or in solitary play, unaware of the actions of other children. Lack of varied, spontaneous make-believe play or social initiative play appropriate to developmental level is also evidenced (see Figure 4.12). Parents of these toddlers may describe them as independent and may be proud of their supposed self-sufficiency. Behavioral symptoms range from mild to severe and disruptive activity may be evidenced. Children are resistant to change in routine,

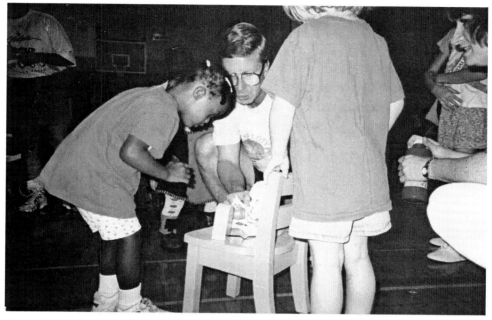

Figure 4.12. Two preschoolers are encouraged by the movement specialist to interact in social play with the toys.

schedule, and activities and these may provoke disruption or aggression. Unprovoked aggressiveness may become a major problem as children become older and larger in physical size (Hagin, 2004).

Communication

Comprehension and the communicative use of speech and gesture are typically deficient in young children with autism. Some children understand little or no language, fail to acquire speech and may remain nonverbal. Less severely affected children have a mixed receptive-expressive disorder, have better comprehension than expression; therefore, their speech is impoverished, poorly articulated, and agrammatical. Other children with autism who speak late may progress rapidly from silence or jargon to fluent, clear, well-formed sentences. These young children may have speech that is literal, repetitive, noncommunicative and is often echolalic. Some of these children speak nonstop to no one in particular in a high-pitched, singsong, or poorly modulated voice and perseverate on favorite topics.

There are various strategies used by speech-language therapists in the remediation of communication disorders. The Tomatis Method (DeJean, 2006) is one method utilized, and is a system of sound stimulation and audio-vocal training. This method aims at improving the functions of the ear and its relationship to listening, understanding and communication. It highlights the importance of the vestibular system in providing the foundation for more complex skills, which is compatible with Sensory Integration theory of Jean Ayres.

Infantile Autism: Early Indicators of Delay

With infants who are labeled as having a developmental delay, there are often behavioral indicators in young infants that may be a clinical sign of undiagnosed autism or PDD. Although there is not one indicator that stands out in the professional's or parent's mind that signifies the child has a problem, upon recalling the developmental history of the child, the parent often recalls child sensitivities to touch, movement, light, or sound which later became more severe and therefore noticeable. They also might recall delays in gestural communication or other symptoms that were not sufficient to cause alarm by the family. The child may present an over or under sensitivity to a specific sensory system, but actually will require respective increased or decreased sensory input to remediate the delay. Proper sensory input is required for optimal behavioral responses. Early intervention programs that highlight sensory modalities could provide a reawakening of the sensory systems to lessen later delays.

Signs that might be noted by the family or a motor developmental specialist that are indicative of an infant with PDD or autism:

- lack of visual awareness of movement in their environment,
- no gestural or nonverbal aspects of communication,
- no visual tracking skills during informal assessment of eye movements,
- lack of social interaction with parents or motor developmental specialist,
- few imitation behaviors,
- no initiation of play with toys,
- resistance or inappropriate response to changes in the environment or in schedule,
- developmental milestones for communication will not be reached

(cooing and babbling may develop during the first 6 months of life and then will disappear). If spoken language develops, speaking of first words occurs between 2 and 3 years of age. Speech is often high-pitched and will be echolalia rather than creative or spontaneous (Batshaw, 2002).

• increase of stress and behavioral disruptions (i.e. crying, aggression) due to noninteraction with the environment. The tactile, vestibular, auditory, visual, and kinesthetic sensory systems have not provided appropriate feedback to allow the child to plan for appropriate interactions (Cowden, Sayers, & Torrey, 1998).

Sensory Dysfunction

Children with autism have some degree of sensory dysfunction (also referred to as sensory integration dysfunction or sensory defensiveness), and some professionals believe it may actually be the root cause of autism (McMullen, 2002). With sensory dysfunction, a child has a contradictory reaction to particular sensory stimuli, sometimes being hypersensitive and other times oblivious to certain sounds, tactile stimuli, or pain. As described by different researchers, it is a combination of symptoms resulting from aversive responses to nonharmful sensory stimuli (Ruble & Sears, 2001), the overactivation of the protective system (Wilbarger & Wilbarger, 1993), and the inability to process or respond appropriately to incoming sensations (Anderson and Emmons, 1996). Most individuals are aroused by a specific stimuli and then return to "normal" level of arousal. An individual with sensory dysfunction may not return to the "normal" level of arousal or may take more time to return to this baseline level. Therefore, the stimuli have a cumulative effect on the individual, and the stimuli build to a level of intolerance (Wilbarger & Wilbarger, 1993). Children with sensory dysfunction have difficulty making choices and they have low frustration levels.

The cause of sensory dysfunction is unknown, but several reasons being proposed include genetic predisposition, prenatal or perinatal complications, environmental teratogens, and allergies (Anderson & Emmons, 1996). Each sensory system is affected in a specific manner. Within the **tactile system**, hyperresponsiveness is expressed by tactile defensiveness and sensitivity to pain, temperature or air currents. Tactile defensiveness is an overreaction to touch experiences, and is often noticed in a newborn or infant that does not like being held, or by negative reactions to clothing labels, texture, or fabric. A reaction to pain or temperature may be extreme (an itch might feel like fire) or may be expressed by reduced sensitivity (a child may show no reaction to a hot stove). To compensate for the discomfort realized by the tactile input, a child might exhibit the following: head banging, scratching, biting oneself, rubbing against large objects, and so forth. Intervention by a movement specialist that includes body brushing with a soft brush followed by joint compression, body massage, or physical exercise, will calm the tactile defensiveness. However, tickling, a commonly used infant stimulation activity, will increase the defensiveness, and should therefore be avoided.

The **vestibular system** may be underresponsive or underactive, and a child's posture and balance, bilateral coordination, and level of arousal are affected. Posture deviations are not evidenced until a toddler begins walking, whereby extensor muscle tone is lacking to hold the body erect. The child may therefore have difficulty walking or riding a tricycle or bicycle on varied or uneven surfaces (riding over pebbles on a street or cracks in the sidewalk). Poor bilateral coordination is evidenced in an infant's difficulty with cross-lateral creeping, and a preschooler's inability to jump in a coordinated pattern or catch a tossed ball. Level of arousal is demonstrated in hyperactivity and distractibility. Children have difficulty in modulating incoming sensory stimuli and vacillate between defensive/anxious states and dormancy states. Because they cannot organize the stimuli, they are either easily overwhelmed or fail to act. To increase stimulation of the vestibular system, children often exhibit behaviors such as rocking, twirling, and flicking fingers. To assist in remediation of each of these areas (posture and balance, bilateral coordination, and arousal level), aquatics, rocking, rolling, swinging, and preschool music/movement activities can be utilized by the movement specialist.

The **kinesthetic system** coordinates with the vestibular system to maintain muscle tone, execute coordinated movement, and move efficiently through space. Preschool children with kinesthetic difficulties may bump into objects when walking, exert more effort to initiate and sustain movement and may therefore seem unmotivated to engage in physical activity. They may exhibit over or underreaching when stair climbing, playing on playground equipment, and when picking up or mouthing objects. Children engage in self-stimulation by stomping,

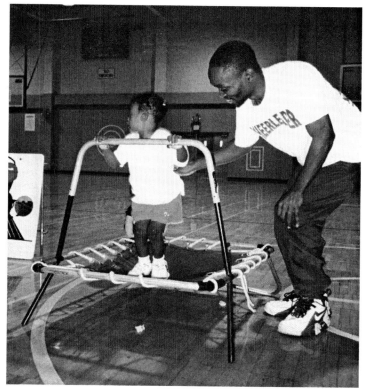

Figure 4.13. This preschooler is engaged in mini tramp jumping while the movement specialist provides physical support and encourages visual attention to the activity.

hand flapping, toe walking, jumping, biting, and head banging. The movement specialist can address intervention through pushing heavy objects, mini-tramp jumping, mirror exercises/activities, therapy ball activities, etc.

The **auditory system** is affected by the volume, pitch, and vibration of the sound as a child receives and differentiates auditory sounds. Loud sounds such as fire alarms, other children crying or yelling, and background noise present problems for the child with autism. Some children simply "shut down" and appear not to hear, while others scream and act out, in order to avoid the overload of auditory input. Preschool children may have difficulty distinguishing speech sounds. For the movement specialist, knowledge about difficulty processing auditory stimuli is critical for planning the intervention environment and providing teaching directions. Quiet areas, free from distraction and outside noise, calm voice, and simple directions should be utilized.

Within the **visual system**, individuals with autism exhibit visual defensiveness (over sensitivity to light), visual overload (inability to recognize things they are looking at even though the child knows the objects), visual distractions (inability to attend to more than one stimuli at a time), and visual sensitivity (glaring lights or eye contact with an adult or other child). Behavior difficulties often occur due to over stimulation of the visual system. The movement specialist must be aware of the visual stimuli within the intervention environment that will affect the child with autism. Avoiding fluorescent lights, teaching in a visually limited environment, not requiring eye-contact, and concern for light glare are a few examples that address the child's visual system limitations.

The **oral** and **olfactory** systems are affected in young children with autism; however, they will not be discussed in detail because they are not primarily addressed within the teaching framework of the motor specialist. It is interesting to note that a connection was found between a child's high mouth palate, poor posture and shallow breathing (Oetter, Frick, & Richter, 1994). In this case, movement efficiency and performance of motor skills might be affected.

This section of the chapter considered the causes of PDD and ASD and the relationship of these disorders to the developmental domains of the young child. Although the domains and the sensory systems of the young child with ASD may be significantly affected, the qualities of children with this disorder vary greatly. Some young children will function much like a child who is typical, and therefore, some of the qualities discussed in this section will not be evidenced. Yet, it is critical that the movement specialist work with other specialists in designing an intervention program that is appropriate for each individual young child. The sensory systems of the young child with ASD may be dramatically affected, and the motor activities to remediate the sensory systems can be utilized in intervention. The movement specialist plays a critical role when working with a child with ASD.

TEAM DECISION-MAKING PROCESS

For infants with medical conditions, a team approach is often critical to the child's survival. Many states require a team approach to multidiciplinary evaluations to determine whether a child qualifies for services due to developmental delay. A multidisciplinary or cross-disciplinary approach enhances intervention services due to collaboration among professionals with specific expertise in various disciplines. Although the team will vary depending on the needs of the child and family/caregivers, a family service coordinator, a family member (or caregiver), and service provider(s) are required team members according to federal legislation, IDEA. Other team members may include, but are not limited to, physicians, nurses, a social worker, physical and occupational therapists, a social worker, a speech language pathologist, a feeding specialist, and an early intervention instruction specialist. A moveement specialist may also be part of the instructional team. Members of the team need to coordinate care for the young child in cooperation with the family. Family and cultural values need to be respected by professionals and remain central in the decision-making process.

Although each professional has an established role dictated by his or her profession, the best services are often provided when roles and responsibilities are flexible and shared among members from the various disciplines. The **transdisciplinary or cross-disciplinary** approach provides holistic management and intervention with the young child. A primary interventionist is responsible for all intervention goals (Howard et al., 1997), while other team members provide input during assessment and intervention through modeling, feedback, or consultation. Utilization of a transdisciplinary or cross-disciplinary approach may therefore decrease the number of professionals, often overwhelming to the family, that are involved in providing services to a young child. Families can work with the primary interventionist while remaining the primary decision maker in the care of their child. This approach may not be appropriate for use within the hospital setting or within some early intervention settings. Therefore an **interdisciplinary** approach might be utilized to facilitate communication and coordination among professionals and with the family. Although assessment may be completed by each professional in isolation, the professionals determine whether the child qualifies for early intervention services through team collaboration. This approach emphasizes professionals sharing assessment information to determine common, integrated programming and intervention goals. Intervention is implemented by each professional in his or her own discipline.

SUMMARY

With advancements in medical technology, many newborns are surviving illnesses and conditions that previously have been fatal. It is necessary for early intervention and motor development professionals, including adapted physical educators, to have knowledge concerning medical terms and conditions in order to provide services to young children and to communicate with families and other professionals. This chapter provided an awareness of eligibility components that may be specified by various states in accordance with IDEA. Working collaboratively with other professionals is critical in evaluation and provision of services.

REFERENCES

Able-Boone, H. (1993). Ethical principles relative to high-technology medicine. In M. Krajicek and R. Tompkins (Eds.) *The medically fragile infant.* Austin, TX: Pro-Ed.

American Academy of Pediatrics Committee on Genetics (1994). Health guidelines for children with Down syndrome. *Pediatrics, 93,* 855–859.

American Psychiatric Association (1994). *Diagnostic and Statistical Manual of Mental Disorders,* 4th ed. (DSM-IV). Washington, DC: American Psychiatric Association.

Anderson, A., & Emmons, P. (1996). *Unlocking the mysteries of sensory dysfunction.* Arlington, TX: Future Horizons.

Apgar, V. (1953). A proposal for a new method of evaluation of the newborn infant. *Current Researches in Anesthesia and Analgesia, 32,* 260–267.

Autism Society of America (2006). *Facts and Statistics.* Retrieved September 29, 2006, from http://www.autism-society.org

Bailey, D., & Wolery, M. (1992). *Teaching infants and preschoolers with disabilities* (2nd ed.). New York: Macmillan.

Barnhart, H. X., Caldwell, M. B., Thomas, P., Mascola, L., Ortiz, I., Hsu, H. W., Schulte, J., Parrott, R., Maldonado, Y., Byers, R., & the Pediatric Spectrum of Disease Clinical Consortium. (1996). Natural history of human immunodeficiency virus disease in perinatally infected children: An analysis from the pediatric spectrum of disease project. *Pediatrics, 97* (5), 710–716.

Baron-Cohen, S., Allen, J., & Gillberg, C. (1992). Can autism be detected at 18 months? The needle, the haystack, and the CHAT. *British Journal of Psychiatry, 161,* 839–843.

Batshaw, M. (Ed.). (1993). The child with developmental disabilities. *Pediatric Clinics of North America, 40* (3). Special issue.

Batshaw, M. L. (Ed.) (2002). *Children with disabilities* (5th ed.) Baltimore: Paul H. Brookes.

Bayley, N. (2006). *Bayley Scales of Infant and Toddler Development* (2nd ed.). San Antonio, TX: Harcourt.

Belman, A. L., Muenz, L. R., Marcus, J. C., Goedert, J. J., Landesman, S., Rubinstein, A., Goodwin, S., Durako, S., & Willoughby, A. (1996). Neurologic status of human immunodeficiency virus 1-infected infants and their controls: A prospective study from birth to 2 years. *Pediatrics, 98* (6), 1109–1118.

Belmonte, M. K., Allen, G., Beckel-Mitchener, A., Boulanger, L. M., Carper, R. A., & Webb, S. J. (2004). Autism and abnormal development of brain connectivity. *The Journal of Neuroscience, 24*(42), 9228–9231.

Blackman, J. A. (1997). *Medical aspects of developmental disablities in children birth to three.* Gaithersburg, MD: Aspen.

Blaxill, M. F. (2004). *What's going on? The question of time trends in autism.* U.S. Department of Health and Human Services; Public Health Reports, 119:536–551.

Boppana, S. B., Fowler, K. B., Vaid, Y., Hedlund, G., Stagno, S., Britt, W. J., & Pass, R. F. (1997). Neuroradiographic findings in the newborn period and long-term out come in children with symptomatic congential cytomegalovirus infection. *Pediatrics, 99* (3), 409–414.

Brann, A. (1985). Factors during neonatal life that influence brain disorders. In J. Freeman (Ed.), *Prenatal and perinatal factors associated with brain disorders* (NIH Publication No. 85-1149, pp. 263–358). Washington, DC: U.S. Department of Health and Human Services.

Brazelton, T. B. (1984). *Neonatal Behavioral Assessment Scale* (2nd ed.). Philadelphia: J. B. Lippincott.

Brunquell, P. J. (1994). Listening to epilepsy. *Infants and Young Children, 7* (1), 24–33.

Bryson, S. E., & Smith, I. M. (1998) Epidemiology of autism: Prevalence, associated characteristics, and implications for research and service delivery. *Mental Retardation and Developmental Disabilities Research Reviews, 4,* 97–103.

Carper, R., & Courchesne, E. (2005). Localized enlargement of the frontal lobe in autism. *Biological Psychiatry, 57,* 126–133.

Chakrabarti, S., & Fombonne, E. (2005). Pervasive developmental disorders in preschool children: Confirmation of high prevalence. *American Journal of Psychiatry, 62*(6). 1133–41.

Charman, T. (2002). The prevalence of autism spectrum disorders. *European Child & Adolescent Psychiatry, 11,* 249–256.

Christiansen, E., Houmann, T., Landorph, S. L., & Skovgaard, A. M. (2006). Assessment and classification of psychopathology in epidemiological research of children 0–3 years of age: A review of the literature. *European Child and Adolescent Psychiatry, 13*(6), 337–346.

Church, E., & Glennen, S. (1992). *Handbook of assistive technology.* San Diego, CA: Singular.

Churchland, P. S. (1986). *Neurophilosophy: Toward a unified science of the mind/brain.* Cambridge, MA: MIT Press.

Clark, R. H., Dykes, F. D., Bachman, T. E., & Ashurst, J. T. (1996). Interventricular hemorrhage and high-frequency ventilation: A meta analysis of prospective clinical trials. *Pediatrics, 98* (6), 1058–1061.

Cohen, W. I. (Ed). (1996, June). Health care guidelines for individuals with Down syndrome. *Down Syndrome Quarterly* [On-line serial, 1(2). Available E-mail: thios@denison.edu.

Coles, C., Smith, I., Fernhoff, P., & Falek, A. (1985). Neonatal neurobehavioral characteristics as correlates of maternal alcohol use during gestation. *Alcoholism, 9,* 454–459.

Corey, L., & Spear, P. G. (1986a). Infections of herpes simplex viruses (Part I). *New England Journal of Medicine, 314* (11), 686–691.

Corey, L., & Spear, P. G. (1986b). Infections of herpes simplex viruses (Part 2). *New England Journal of Medicine, 314* (12), 749–757.

Covington, C., Nordstrom-Klee, B., Ager, J., Sokol, R., & Delaney-Black, V. (2002). Birth to age 7 growth of children prenatally exposed to drugs: A prospective cohort study. *Neurotoxicology and Teratology, 24,* 489–496.

Cowan, J. J., Hellman, D., & Chudwin, D. (1984). Maternal transmission of acquired immune deficiency syndrome. *Pediatrics, 73,* 382–386.

Cowden, J., Sayers, K., & Torrey, C. (1998). *Pediatric adapted motor development and exercise.* Springfield, IL: Charles C Thomas.

Dejean, V. (2006). *Tomatis, autism, and sensory integration.* New York: Spectrum Center.

DiCicco-Bloom, E., Lord, C., Zwaigenbaum, L., Courchesne, E., Dager, S. T., Schmitz, C., Schultz, R. T., Crawley, J., & Young, L. J. (2006). The developmental neurobiology of autism spectrum disorder. *The Journal of Neuroscience, 26*(26), 6897–6906.

Dunn, J. M., & Leitschuh, C. (2006). *Special physical education* (8th ed.). Dubuque, IA: Kendall/Hunt.

Dykens, E. M., Hodappp, R. M., Ort, S. I., & Leckman, J. F. (1993). Trajectory of adaptive behavior in males with fragile X sydrome. *Journal of Autism and Developmental Disorders, 23,* 135–145.

Enhorning, G., Shennan, A., & Possmayer, F. (1985). Prevention of respiratory distress syndrome by tracheal installation of surfactant: A randomized clinical trial. *Pediatrics, 76,* 145–153.

Ensher, G. L., & Clark, D. A. (1994). *Newborns at risk: Medical care and psychoeducational intervention* (2nd ed.). Gaithersburg, MD: Aspen.

Fishler, K., & Koch, R. (1991). Mental development in Down syndrome mosaicism. *American Journal of Mental Deficiency, 96,* 345–351.

Folstein, S. E., & Rosen-Heidley, B. (2001). Genetics of autism: Complex aetiology for a heterogeneous disorder. *Nature Reviews Genetics 2*(12), 943–955.

Fombonne, E. (2003). Epidemiological surveys of autism and other pervasive developmental disorders: An update. *Journal of Autism and Developmental Disorders, 33*(4), 365–382.

Frank, D. A., Augustyn, M., Knight, W. G., Pell, T., & Zuckerman, B. (2001). Growth, development, and behavior in early childhood following prenatal cocaine exposure. *Journal of the American Medical Association, 285*(12), 1613–1625.

Fredrick, J. (1973). Epilepsy and pregnancy: A report from the Oxford Record Linkage Study. *British Medical Journal, 2,* 442.

Garron, D. (1977). Intelligence among persons with Turner's Syndrome. *Behavorial*

Genetics, 7, 105–127.

Gilman, S., & Newman, S. W. (1992). *Essentials of clinical neuroanatomy and neurophysiology* (8th ed.). Philadelphia: F.A. Davis.

Gonik, B., & Hammill, H. A. (1990). AIDS in pregnancy. *Seminars in Pediatric Infectious Disease, 1,* 82–88.

Graham, R. B. (1990). *Physiological psychology.* Belmont: CA.

Hagin, R. A. (2004). Autism and other severe pervasive developmental disorders. In F. M. Kline and L. B. Silver (Eds.) *The educators guide to mental health issues in the classroom* (pp. 55–73). Baltimore: Brookes.

Handler, A. S., Mason, E. D., Rosenberg, D. L., & Davis, F. G. (1994). The relationship between exposure during pregnancy to cigarette smoking and cocaine use and placenta previa. *American Journal of Obstetrics and Gynecology, 170* (3), 884–889.

Hanshaw, H. B., Dudgeon, J. A., & Marshall, W. C. (1985). *Viral diseases of the fetus and newborn.* Philadelphia: W.B. Saunders.

Hazlett, H. C., Poe, M., Gerig, G., Smith, R. G., Provenzale, J., Ross, A., Gilmore, J., & Piven, J. (2005). Magnetic resonance imaging and head circumference study of brain size in autism: Birth through age 2 years. *Archives of General Psychiatry, 62,* 1366–1376.

Hitti, M. WebMDHealth. *Morbidity and Mortality Weekly Report: Surveillance Summaries;* February 9, 2007; vol. 56: pp. 1–40.

Hoshino, Y., Yashima, Y., Ishige, K., Tachibana, R., Watanabe, M., Kaneko, M., & Kumashiro, H. (1980). An epidemiological study of autistic children in Fukushima-ken. *Japan Journal of Child Psychiatry, 21*(2), 111–128.

Howard, V. F., Williams, B. F., Port, P. D., & Lepper, C. (1997). *Very young children with special needs: A formative approach for the 21st century.* Upper Saddle River, NJ: Prentice-Hall.

Johnson, R. C., & Abelson, R. B. (1969). Intellectual behavioral, and physical characteristics associated with trisomy, translocation, and mosaic types of Down syndrome. *American Journal of Mental Deficiency 73* (6), 852 855.

Jones, K. L. (1997). *Smith's recognizable patterns of human malformation* (5th ed.). Philadelphia: W. B. Saunders Co.

Jones, A., Cork, C., & Chowdhury, U. (2006). Autism spectrum disorders 1: Presentation and assessment. *Community Practitioner, 79*(3), 97–98.

Juul-Dam, N., Townsend, J., & Courchesne, E. (2001). Prenatal, perinatal and neonatal factors in autism, pervasive developmental disorder-not otherwise specified, and the general population. *Pediatrics, 107*(4), E63.

Kanner, L. (1943). Autistic disturbances of affective contact. *Nervous Child, 2,* 217–250.

Kennelly, C. (1990). Tracheostomy care: Parents as learners. *American Journal of Maternal and Child Nursing, 12,* 264–267.

Kettrick, R. G., & Donar, M. E. (1985). The ventilator-dependent child: Medical and social care. *Critical Care: State of the Art, 6,* 1–38.

Koller, H., Lawson, K., Rose, S. A., Wallace, I., & McCarton, C. (1997). Patterns of cognitive development in very low birth weight children during the first six years of life. *Pediatrics, 99* (3), 383–389.

Kugelman, A., Durand, M., & Garg, M. (1997). Pulmonary effect of inhaled furosemide in ventilated infants with severe bronchopulmonary dysplasia. *Pediatrics, 99* (1), 71–75.

Kuntz, K. R. (1996). Medical and nursing issues. In L. A. Kurtz, P. W. Dowrick, S. E. Levy, & M. L. Batshaw (Eds.), *Handbook of developmental disabilities: Resources for interdisciplinary care* (pp. 342–448). Gaithersburg, MD: Aspen.

Kurtz, L. A., Dowrick, P. W, Levy, S. E., & Batshaw, M. L. (1996). *Handbook of developmental disabilities: Resources for interdisciplinary care.* Gaithersburg, MD: Aspen.

Kutscher M., Attwood, T., & Wolff, R. (2005). *Kids in the Syndrome Mix of ADHD, LD, Asperger's, Tourette's, Bipolar and More! The One Stop Guide for Parents, Teachers, and Other Professionals.* London: Jessica Kingsley Publishers.

Kwiatkowski, D. J., & Short, M. P. (1994). Tuberous sclerosis. *Archives of Dermatology, 130,* 348–354.

Lee, R. V. (1988). Parasites and pregnancy: The problems of malaria in toxoplasmosis. *Clinics in Perinatology, 15,* 351–364.

Levitt, S. (1982). *Treatment of cerebral palsy and motor delay.* Palo Alto, CA: Blackwell Scientific.

Lichtenstein, M. A. (1986). Pediatric home tracheostomy care: A parent's guide. *Pediatric Nursing, 12,* 41–48, 69.

Louch, G. (1993). Chronic lung disease. In M. Krajicek & R. Tompkins (Eds), *The medically fragile infant.* Austin, TX: Pro-ed.

Luiselli, J. K., & Luiselli, T. E. (1995). A behavior analysis approach toward chronic food refusal in children with gastrostomy-tube dependency. *Topics in Early Childhood Special Education, 15* (1), 1–18.

Manjiviona, J., & Prior, M. (1995). Comparison of Asperger syndrome and high-functioning autistic children on a test of motor impairment. *Journal of Autism and Developmental Disorders, 25*(1), 23–39.

McCarton, C. M., Wallace, I. F, Divon, M., & Vaughan, H. G. (1996). Cognitive and neurologic development of the premature, small for gestational age infant through age 6: Comparison by birth weight and gestational age. *Pediatrics, 98* (6), 1167–1178.

McMullen, P. (2002). Living with sensory dysfunction in autism. In R.A. Huebner (Ed.), *Autism: A sensorimotor approach to management.* Aspen: Gaithersburg, MD.

Meadow, S. R. (1968). Anticonvulsant drugs and congenital abnormalities. *Lancet, 2,* 1296.

MedlinePlus (2005). Small for gestational age (SGA). Retrieved February 17, 2006, from http://www.nlm.nih.gov/medlineplus/ency/article/002302.htm.

Miller, L., & Lane, S. J. (2000). Toward a consensus in terminology in sensory integrative theory, and practice: Part I: Taxonomy of neurophysiological processes. *Sensory Integration Special Interest Section Quarterly, 23,* 1–4.

Miller-Loncar, C., Lester, B., Seifer, R., Lagasse, L., Bauer, C., & Shankaran, S. (2005). Predictors of motor development in children prenatally exposed to cocaine. *Neurotoxicology and Teratology, 27*(2), 213–220.

Mok, J. Q., Giaquinto, C., & DeRossi, A. (1987). Infants born to mothers seropositive for human immunodeficiency virus: Preliminary finds from a multicenter

European study. *Lancet, 21,* 1164–1168.

Mooney, E. L., Gray, K. M., & Tonge, B. J., (2006). Early features of autism: Repetitive behaviours in young children. *European Child & Adolescent Psychiatry, 15*(1), 12–18.

Narbarro, D. (1954). *Congenital syphillis.* London: E. Arnold.

National Center for Clinical Infant Programs (1995). *Diagnostic Classification of Mental Health and Developmental Disorders of Infancy and Early Childhood.* Arlington, VA: Zero to Three/National Center for Clinical Infant Programs, 2000 14th Street North, Suite 380.

National Center on Physical Activity and Disability (NCPAD) (2004). *Spina bifida– Physical activity guidelines fact sheet.* Retrieved at www.ncpad.org.

Nemours Foundation (2006). *Spina Bifida.* Retrieved on September 16, 2006 from http://www.kidshealth.org/parent/system/ill/spina_bifida.html.

Oetter, P., Frick, S., & Richter, E. (1994). *Oral motor function and its relationship to development and treatment.* Hugo, MN: PDP Press.

Papille, L., Munsick-Bruno, G., & Schaefer, A. (1983). Relationship of cerebral interventricular hemorrhage and early childhood neurologic handicaps. *Journal of Pediatrics, 103,* 273–277.

Peterson, N. L. (1987). *Early intervention for handicapped and at risk children.* Denver, CO: Love.

Pueschel, S. (Ed.). (1978). *Down syndrome: Growing and learning.* Kansas City, KS: Andrews & McMeel.

Robins, D. L., Fein, D., Barton, M. L., & Green, J. A. (2001). Modified Checklist for Autism in Toddlers (M-CHAT). *Journal of Autism and Developmental Disorders, 31*(2), 131–144.

Ruble, L. A., & Sears, L. L. (2001). The Development of autism: A self regulatory perspective. *Journal of Autism and Developmental Disorders, 31*(5), 471–482.

Santos, K. E. (1992). Fragile X syndrome: An educator's role in identification, prevention, and intervention. *Remedial and Special Education, 13,* 32–39.

Scafidi, F. A., Field, T. M., Wheeden, A., Schanberg, S., Kuhn, C., Symanski, R., Zimmerman, E., & Bandstra, E. S. (1996). Cocaine-exposed preterm neonates show behavioral and hormonal differences. *Pediatrics, 97* (6), 851–855.

Scherzer, A. L., & Tscharnuter, I. (1990). *Early diagnosis and therapy in cerebral palsy: A primer on infant developmental problems* (2nd ed., rev., expanded). New York: Marcel Dekker.

Schumann, C. M., Hamstrea, J., Goodlin-Jones, B. L., Lotspeich, L. J., Kwon, H., & Buonocore, M. H. (2004). The amygdale is enlarged in children but not adolescents with autism: The hippocampus is enlarged at all ages. *Journal of Neuroscience, 24,* 6392–6401.

Shankaran, S., Das, A., Bauer, C., Bada, H., Lester, B., & Wright, L. (2004). Association between patterns of maternal substance use and infant birth weight, length, and head circumference. *Pediatrics, 114*(2), 226–234.

Sherrill, C. (2004). *Adapted physical activity, recreation, and sport: Crossdisciplinary and lifespan* (6th ed.). New York: McGraw-Hill.

Sindel, B. D., Maisels, M. J., & Ballantine, T. V. (1989). Gastroesophageal reflux to the proximal esophagus in infants with bronchopulmonary dysplasia. *American Journal of Disease of Children, 143,* 1103–1106.

Singer, L. T., Arendt, R., Minnes, S., Farkas, K., Salvator, A., & Kirchner, H. L. (2002). Cognitive and motor outcomes of cocaine-exposed infants. *JAMA, 287,* 1952–1960.

Singer, L. T., Garber, R., & Kliegman, R. (1991). Neurobehavioral sequelae of fetal cocaine exposure. *Journal of Pediatrics, 119,* 667–672.

Sontag, S. J. (1990) The medical management of reflux esophagitis: Role of antacids and acid inhibition. *Gastroenterology Clinics of North America, 19,* 683–712.

Stagno, S., & Whitley, R. (1985). Herpes virus infections of pregnancy: Part I: Cytomegalovirus and Epstein-Barr virus infections. *New England Journal of Medicine, 313* (20), 1271.

Starrett, A. (1991). Growth in developmental disabilities. In A. J. Capute & P. J. Accardo (Eds.). *Developmental disabilities in infancy and childhood* (pp. 181–187). Baltimore: Paul H. Brookes.

Stromland, K., & Hellstrom, A. (1996). Fetal alcohol syndrome: An ophthalmological and socioeducational perspective study. *Pediatrics, 97* (6), 845–855.

Sugie, Y., Sugie, H., Fukuda, T., & Ido, M. (2005). Neonatal factors in infants with autistic disorder and typically developing infants. *Autism: The International Journal of Research and Practice, 9*(5), 487–494.

Swayze, V. W., Johnson, V. P., Hanson, J. W., Piven, J., Sato, Y., Giedd, J. N., Mosnik, D., & Andreasen, N. E. (1997). Magnetic resonance imaging of brain anomalies in fetal alcohol syndrome. *Pediatrics, 99* (2) 232–240.

Tarr, P. I., Hass, J. E., & Christie, D. L. (1996). Biliary atresia, cytomegalovirus, and age at referral. *Pediatrics, 97* (6) 828–831.

Thommessen, J., Kase, B. F., Riis, G., & Heiberg, A. (1991). The impact of feeding problems on growth and energy intake in children with cerebral palsy. *European Journal of Clinical Health, 45,* 479–487.

Thompson, E. (1989). A genetics primer for early service providers. *Infants and Young Children, 2* (1) 37–48.

Thurman, S. K, & Widerstrom, A. H. (1990). *Infants and young children with special needs.* Baltimore: Paul H. Brookes.

Trillingsgaard, A., Sorensen, E. U., Nemec, G., & Jorgensen, M. (2005). What distinguishes autism spectrum disorders from other developmental disorders before the age of four years? *European Child & Adolescent Psychiatry, 14,* 65–72.

Turnell, W. (1993). Omphalocele and gastroschisis. In K. W. Ashcraft and T. M. Holder (Eds.), *Pediatric Surgery* (pp. 546–556).

Van Deusen, J. & Brunt, D. (1997). *Assessment in occupational therapy and physical therapy.* Philadelphia: W. B. Saunders.

Vaughn, B., & Goldberg, S. (1994). Quality of toddler-mother attachment in children with Down syndrome: Limits to interpretation of strange situation behavior. *Child Development, 65,* 96–108.

Westman, J. C. (1990). *Handbook of learning disabilities: A multisystem approach.* Boston: Allyn & Bacon.

Widerstrom, A., Mowder., B., & Sandall, S. (1991). *At-risk and handicapped newborns and infants.* Englewood Cliffs. NJ: Prentice-Hall.

Wilbarger, P., & Wilbarger, J. (1991). *Sensory defensiveness in children aged 2–12: An intervention guide for parents & caretakers.* Oak Park Heights, MN: PDP Press.

Wilbarger, P., & Wilbarger, J. (1993). *Sensory defensiveness and related social/emotional and neurological problems.* Professional development programs workshop in Albuquerque, NM.

Williams, J., & Brayne, C. (2006). Screening for autism spectrum disorders. *Autism, 10*(1). 11–35.

Wing, L., & Potter, D. (2002). The epidemiology of autistic spectrum disorders: Is the prevalence rising? *Mental Retardation and Developmental Disabilities Research Reviews, 8,* 151–161.

Wolff, R. (2006). *More Autism Information.* Retrieved on September 30, 2006 from http://www.pediatricneurology.com/autism.htm.

Chapter 5

ASSESSMENT

Chapter Objectives: After studying this chapter, the reader will be able to:
1. Define assessment;
2. Discuss the role of the motor specialist in a team approach to assessment;
3. Discuss the ROADMAP Model to understand the process of assessment;
4. Discuss the major purposes of assessment and distinguish among the various assessment procedures;
5. Describe and use various assessment instruments appropriate for young children.

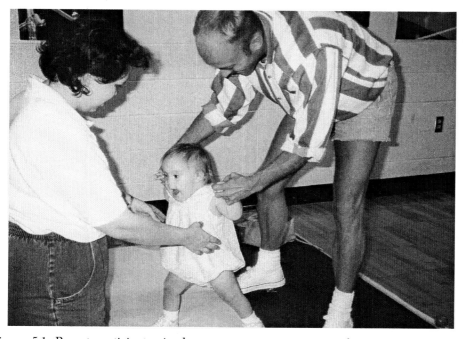

Figure 5.1. Parent participates in the assessment process, providing motivation to her child.

"Learning to move and moving to learn" is a phrase that many movement specialists and physical educators incorporate into their educational philosophy. Teachers of infants and young children with delay/disability understand the relationship between movement and learning: children attain voluntary actions and then use a particular action to facilitate learning in other domains. Actions communicate thoughts and movement throughout one's environment, thereby enhancing one's development. Due to professionals' personal beliefs concerning the importance of movement, teachers are highly motivated to engage students in gross motor activities, but frequently ignore appropriate assessment of young children's motor abilities. Teachers feel that time constraints do not allow for lengthy assessments or for more than one assessment period; however each could increase the reliability and validity of the results. Therefore, to best facilitate student progress and success, to utilize the student's best effort and to maximize student capabilities, it is critical to continuously assess infants and young children. Assessment can be completed for various purposes and therefore several procedures must be available for the movement specialist.

Assessment can be defined as any activity designed to elicit accurate and reliable sample behaviors of infants and young children. As a result of the behavior exhibited by the child, inferences relative to developmental skill status along a continuum can be made (Rossetti, 1990). Assessment may be formal using standardized, norm-referenced, or criterion-referenced instruments, or informal using developmental observational checklists or profiles (see Figure 5.2). Determination of eligibility for special education services can be addressed and the areas for remediation and methods of intervention identified.

Assessment provides an entry level measurement of the child's skills and desired family outcomes to produce information determining appropriate and relevant intervention goals and objectives (Bricker & Waddell, 2002; Zittel, 1994). Assessment results provide the foundation for appropriate programming, and thus provide the first step in successful intervention (Auxter, Pyfer, & Huetig, 2005; Horvat & Kalakian, 1996). This process should be continuous, comprehensive, cooperative, and coordinated. Observations, caregiver interviews and questionnaires, as well as other informal assessment techniques are part of this process. Although one of the primary objectives of the movement specialist may be to administer a specific assessment instru-

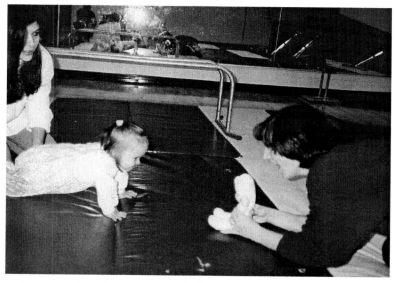

Figure 5.2. The caregiver is engaged with the movement specialist during curriculum-based assessment.

ment, it is necessary to interpret the child's total behavior throughout the entire assessment process. It is critical that the movement specialist cultivate his or her observation skills, for as Greenspan (1992) stated, "A test is no more valid than one's observations."

The assessment of infants, toddler, and preschoolers is only useful if it provides answers to significant questions such as:

1. Does the assessment process provide information that directs eligibility, placement, and intervention?
2. Does the process provide information that is useful to families and program providers? (Auxter, Pyfer, & Huettig, 2005)
   Additionally, it is critical that one considers the following questions:
3. Is the assessment process appropriate for the chronological age and developmental level of the child?
4. Does the process provide appropriate opportunities for the child with specific disabilities to demonstrate his/her capabilities?
5. Do the instruments encompass an age range that allows the evaluator to determine specific functional skills of the child with a disability across age levels?
6. Is the process teacher, family, and child friendly?

TEAM APPROACH

It is necessary to utilize a multidisciplinary, interdisciplinary, trans-disciplinary, or cross-disciplinary approach to assessment because assessment is a complex process used to determine relative strengths and weaknesses of the child in all domains (cognitive, psychomotor, and social-emotional). The movement specialist should determine eligibility of young children or plan for intervention with other professionals and the child's family (see Figure 5.3).

Confusion exists among professionals regarding the use of terminology describing team approaches (multidisciplinary, interdisciplinary, transdisciplinary, or cross-disciplinary). Members of multidisciplinary teams perform assessments independent of one another, have very little collaboration, and view their specific roles as separate from the other disciplines. They do not assist each other in determining specific goals for a child's program. Members of interdisciplinary teams develop collaborative goals and individual service plans. According to Howard, Williams, Port, and Lepper (1997), there should be "three

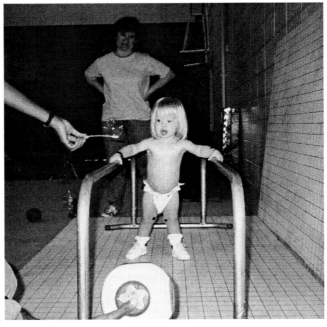

Figure 5.3. The presence and influence of the child's family increases the validity and reliability of the assessment.

commitments in an interdisciplinary team model: a unified service plan, decision making as a group, and the opportunity to interact across many disciplines" (p. 417). Transdisciplinary teams encourage a role sharing approach to intervention; however, with highly coordinated efforts, one or two team members are responsible for the implementation of the actual intervention goals. **Arena assessment**, an extension of the transdisciplinary model, is often completed for infants and young children when determining eligibility for special education services. One examiner, the facilitator, administers test items while the other team members observe the child's behavior and score their respective instrument protocols (Widerstrom, Mowder, & Sandall, 1991; Wolery & Dyk, 1984). The movement specialist, or an occupational or physical therapist if available, will often serve as the facilitator when the child's major deficit is in the motor domain.

Cross-disciplinary teams is a more accurate descriptor of the professionals and parents who must make "cutting edge" decisions which shape the future as they live each day. Wisdom of individuals from diverse fields is needed to examine different perspectives and integrate content across disciplines and develop a broad theory base for early intervention. The interdisciplinary and transdisciplinary or cross-disciplinary approaches involve cooperation and collaboration with professionals from other disciplines. Each of the models encourages interaction within and across many disciplines. Either of these approaches is recommended during the assessment of young children; however, as reference is made in this text to movement specialist, the term cross-disciplinary will be used as a more progressive descriptor of the broad theory bases involved in determining the child's functioning levels and designing techniques for intervention.

Assessment of motor development is an important component in the evaluation process of young children as movement is closely tied to and interrelated with both perceptual and conceptual development (Horvat, 2003). Within the medical model, assessment of the motor domain has typically been provided for infants by physical and occupational therapists. Given the shortage of these professionals to treat developmental movement needs of infants and young children, the movement specialist, which might be the adapted physical educator, can often be an integral member of the cross-disciplinary team within the educational model. Professionals from the disciplines of adapted physical education and motor development can work effectively in the psychomotor domain with infants and young children with delays or disabilities.

When working with infants or toddlers, the following areas should be addressed: (a) assessment; (b) curriculum sequences in motor development including tone, strength, motor control, and sensory motor development; (c) the utilization of appropriate response contingent toys/materials for sensory stimulation and physical and motor development; (d) strategies for relaxation, socialization and play behavior; and (e) providing families with information, skills, and support related to enhancing the child's physical growth and development. The movement specialist, which may be the adapted physical educator is often the team member who is highly knowledgeable of the developmental motor areas and can be most responsible for providing appropriate assessment. When the services of an occupational or physical therapist are available team coordination is essential. Each member has different expertise and a slightly different emphasis in assessment and programming which can be shared collaboratively (Cowden & Eason, 1991).

ROADMAP MODEL

One of the greatest challenges of performing an appropriate assessment of young children is to determine exactly what steps should be taken to perform the assessment. The ROADMAP Model (Role of Assessment Directed Movements, Actions, and Patterns) (Cowden & Torrey, 1995) (see Figure 5.4) provides a plan of action and framework for performing assessments of young children. It identifies "inputs," "processes," "products," "outputs," and "outcomes" that must be addressed through the assessment process to meet the needs of the child and family. The entire model depicts the involvement of the movement specialist in the assessment process when determining eligibility for services. However, for use in developing appropriate movement programs, the movement specialist most typically is involved in the first three components of the model.

"Inputs" provide information prior to the assessment situation. The assessment team (which includes the young child's family) gathers information on the history of the child and family to determine the direction of assessment, instrumentation, and team composition. **"Processes"** involve formal testing as well as informal observations relative to the child's health and emotional well-being, social interac-

ROADMAP

Family Service Coordinator
Adapted Motor Developmentalist
Related Services
Speech & Language

CHILD
FAMILY
Assessment Team

Physician
Psychologist
Assessment Teacher
Special Education Teacher

ARENA ASSESSMENT

INPUTS	PROCESSES		PRODUCTS	OUTPUTS	OUTCOMES
Medical history	**Initial contact**	**Gross motor patterns**	**Foundation for intervention**	**Appropriate programming**	**Maximize development**
Prenatal	Health status	Cephalocaudal	Inferences for programs	Status quo home with	Normalization
Birth	Emotional status	Proximodistal	Individualization	caregiver	Prevention of secondary
Hospital	Family data	Rolling	Continued monitoring	Placement	disability
Sensory data	Family concerns	Prone crawl	Family awareness of child's needs	Home based	Accountability
Family considerations	Environmental responses	Quadruped crawl	Family service coordination	Center based	Financial burden decreased
Teaming considerations	Child-caregiver considerations	Supine tuck	Prioritization of needs	Alternative programs	Increased family and
Instrument selection	**Informal–free play observations**	Bilateral-unilateral	Establishing goals	Coordination with other	community awareness
Review of instrument	Alertness/awareness	Airplane position	Establish IFSP/IEP	agencies	Maintenance of LRE
Multicultural concerns	Determine tonicity	Rhythm	Identification of sensory &	Minimization of cost	Transition
Time considerations	Primitive reflex patterns	Sitting/standing postures	learning strengths	Social play and recreation	Generalization of learned
Materials needed	Analysis of sensory systems	Walking/gait analysis	Teaching/intervention	Social interaction	skills
Facility concerns	Equilibrium reactions/balance	Locomotor patterns	Joint goal setting	Physical & health	
Legal issues	Functional mobility	**Fine motor/hand function**	Consultation	management	
Organization	Gross motor patterns	Grasp reflex	Identification of physical needs		
Financial resources	Visual pursuits	Grasping	Adaptive equipment		
Right to services	Fine motor/hand function	Reaching	Family directed service delivery		
	Social interactive signals	Releasing			
	Child caregiver interactions	Stacking			
	Environment interactions	Copying forms			
	Interest for toys	Eye hand coordination			
	Play	Object control			
	Formal testing	**Closure/wrap-up**			
	Tonicity	Closing parent interview			
	Reflex patterns	Representativeness of child's performance			
	Analysis of sensory systems	Brief summary of child's performance			
	Equilibrium and balance	Referrals			
	Functional mobility	Parent concerns			

Figure 5.4. The Roadmap model details the assessment process and role of the cross-disciplinary assessment team. From "A ROADMAP for assessing infants, toddlers, and preschoolers: The role of the adapted motor developmentalists," by J. E. Cowden and C. C. Torrey, Authors, 1995. *Adapted Physical Activity Quarterly,* 12 (1) p. 6. Copyright 1995 by Human Kinetics Publishers, Inc. Reprinted with permission.

tive signals between the child and caregiver, and child responses to the environment. **"Products"** are the intermediate results of the entire assessment process and establish the foundation for intervention. Results from the actual assessment, combined with input data, allow the assessment team to determine "products" that are relevant to the child and family. Identification of the needs of the child and concerns, priorities, and resources of the family allows for the development of the Individualized Family Service Plan or Individualized Education Plan (IFSP or IEP) (see Figure 5.5). The assessment team prioritizes goals and objectives, identifies teaching and intervention strategies, and identifies program considerations, service delivery, and resources.

"Outputs," the direct results of the assessment process, influence ultimate gains for the child, family, and society. Appropriate placement and programming are obtained, and social play, recreation opportunities, and physical or health management strategies continue to be explored. Coordination with other agencies and cost-effective procedures are outlined. "**Outcomes**" are the final result of the assessment process, and indicate overall gains for the child, family, and society. Ultimately, the child's development is maximized, normalization has been attained, secondary disabilities have been prevented, and financial burden to society has been minimized.

As a member of the cross-disciplinary team, the movement specialist must evaluate the skills of infants and toddlers with multisystem delays or diagnosed disabilities. Emphasis should continue to stress normal developmental processes. Henderson (1994) suggested that theoretical vocabulary is necessary for analyzing and interpreting immature and mature movement patterns. Therefore, the movement specialist must acquire a theoretical background (see Chapter 1) to assist in the evaluation of young children and make critical decisions for determining the child's functioning level in the motor domain (Cowden & Torrey, 1995). The movement specialist establishes an assessment approach based on his or her theoretical frame of reference.

As a member of the cross-disciplinary team, additional competencies are necessary for the movement specialist to adequately function

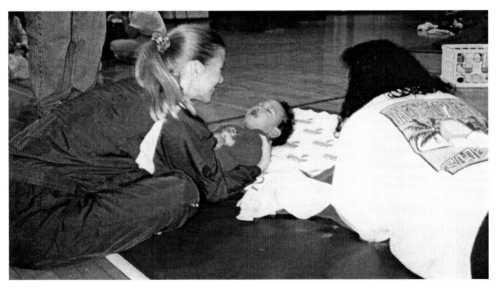

Figure 5.5. Identification of the child's needs and the concerns, priorities, and resources of the family contribute to the development of the IFSP.

within the team framework. Among other competencies, knowledge of data collection options and the limitations of assessment measures are critical. The movement specialist must have the ability to integrate assessment results with members of other disciplines and summarize these into implications and recommendations for content and process of intervention. This chapter provides an overview of instruments available for individuals who conduct assessments in the psychomotor domain.

PURPOSES AND PROCEDURES FOR ASSESSMENT

Assessment is completed for three major purposes: **screening**, determining **eligibility** for special education or medical services, and planning for **educational intervention**. Screening determines which children need further testing by identifying children who are not within normal ranges of development. **Standardized instruments** provide normative data which allow comparisons between children; however, informal checklists and observations may sometimes be utilized. Eligibility for medical or educational services must follow federal or state guidelines and children must often be assessed with instruments that provide standardized test scores. Therefore, a formal, standardized or norm-referenced instrument is often required when determining eligibility for services. The instrument must be more comprehensive than those used for screening. When developmental age ranges are provided in the assessment instrument **criterion tests** are sometimes utilized for determining eligibility for early intervention services. Criterion-referenced tests have historically been used to provide more complete and specific information when program planning is the major objective of the assessment.

Other assessment procedures have emerged and are considered complimentary components of the assessment process. As a member of the cross-disciplinary team, the movement specialist must be aware of the value of these components and be knowledgeable of their use. **Judgment-based assessment** is a formal process of collecting, structuring, and quantifying ideas and observations of professionals and caregivers about child environmental indicators (Neisworth, 1990). **Convergent assessment** is the process that incorporates information from various assessments, sources, occasions, and settings to describe the child's developmental status (Bagnato & Neisworth, 1990). Both of these procedures can be used along with standardized assessment instruments in determining eligibility for services.

Curriculum-based assessment (CBA) is a form of skill appraisal that determines the child's achievement and instructional needs along a continuum of objectives within course content (Bagnato, Neisworth, & Munson, 1989). As implied, this form of assessment is conducted to assist in planning and implementing intervention programs. More recently, **transactional assessment** (Parks, 2006) has become a focus in the assessment of young children. Some components of transactional assessment can be utilized for determining eligibility and for program planning. Transactional assessment involves observation and interview techniques to assess the physical environment and interactions between the child, caregiver, and professional. Factors to assess within the environment include physical space, daily routines, and developmentally appropriate play materials. Interactions include sensitivity to the child's moods or cues and allowances for child and caregiver preferences. The importance of the interactions between the individual and all aspects of his/her respective environment is also supported through the **ecological assessment approach** (see Figure 5.6). Sherrill (1993) stated "ecological theory creates the framework for families and professionals working together and for collaborative models in which many disciplines cooperate" (p. 130). Recently, Sherrill (2004) emphasized the importance of ecosystem changes and supports as important considerations in the assessment process rather than the sole importance of individual differences (disability, characteristics, and unique attributes).

These approaches and other informal measures are increasingly being used by Child Search teams during initial eligibility evaluations of young children and by teachers for program planning. A combination of the transactional and judgment-based approaches have been used effectively at a university-affiliated medical and high-risk infant clinic where time and space are major limitations. The movement specialist observes and assesses the child's abilities while interrelating with the medical team to predict child developmental outcomes (Cowden & Sayers, 1997).

However, the most effective method of assessment must actually incorporate the strengths of each of the types of assessment procedures that have been defined. Another example, a systematic assessment

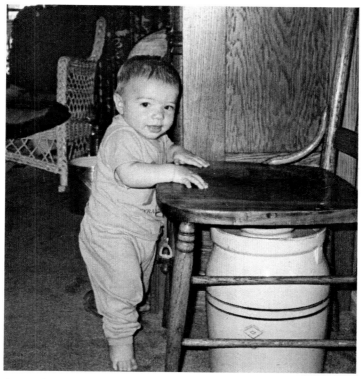

Figure 5.6. An ecological assessment includes interviews and observations of the child's movements and interactions with all aspects of his environment.

process of "head-to-toe" analysis for young children used at the University of New Orleans Adapted Physical Education and Motor Development Clinic, is termed **Progressive Interactive Assessment. Progressive Interactive Assessment** is a concentrated, progressive process which *emphasizes the quality of services to be provided to the child and family* and involves the following components: (a) unified communication between the family/caregiver and cross-disciplinary team members (discontinue old, out-dated "turf" battles among disciplines, for example, adapted physical education, physical and occupational therapy); (b) embedded instrumentation (multiple units and types of assessment, e.g., standardized, criterion-referenced, curriculum-based); (c) continuous examination of physical, biological, cultural, psychological, social-emotional, and cognitive systems; (d) analysis of functional and discriminative movement patterns; (e) action plan or "blueprint" for meaningful system individualization (ever-changing, nonlinear, adaptable); (f) task analysis approach to intervention using both a holistic approach and patterns of interrelationships; (g) use of rigorous methods for research analysis combining qualitative and quantitative approaches when necessary for accurate, reliable, and valid measures of individual changes in response to intervention; (h) accountability, commitment and compromise combined with common sense and wisdom; and (i) integration of strategies or interdependence of all components. Application of these **Progressive Interactive Assessment** components has provided caregivers with opportunities to learn how to implement a home program and is based on qualitative and quantitative methods of inquiry.

Within the three major purposes of assessment, several instruments will be described and critically evaluated (see Table 5.1). The listing of instruments described is not exhaustive; there are many informal methods of assessment that are not included in this chapter. However, instruments which are available nationally for early interventionists are described. The following factors were considered in evaluating instruments: (a) domains assessed, (b) feasibility for administration, (c) thoroughness of the instrument, (d) technical adequacy (when appropriate), (e) adaptations or modifications for various disabilities, (f) the appropriateness of the instrument for specific settings, and (g) examiner qualifications.

Table 5.1. Assessment Instruments for Young Children.

Instruments	Purpose/type of instrument	Age Range	Feasibility
Ages and Stages Questionnaire: A parent-completed, child-monitoring system, Second Edition (Bricker, et al., 1999)	Screening in 5 major developmental areas	4 months–5 years	Low cost, easy and quick to administer. Translations in 3 languages.
Assessment, Evaluation, and Programming System for Infants and Children, Second Edition, (Bricker, 2002)	Criterion referenced, functional skills assessment for individuals with disabilities with corresponding curriculum.	1 month–8 years	Activity based assessment: Motor tasks are not in sequential order.

continued

Table 5.1. Assessment Instruments for Young Children–*Continued.*

Instruments	Purpose/type of instrument	Age Range	Feasibility
Battelle Developmental Inventory, Second Edition (Newborg, 2004)	Evaluation for eligibility: standardized, norm-referenced	0–7.11 years	Timely to administer; however, screening instrument available.
Bayley Scales of Infant and Toddler Development, Third Edition (Bayley, 2006)	Evaluation of infants and young children: standardized and norm-referenced	1–42 months	Directions are easily understood but specific procedures must be followed. Accommodations, but not modifications are allowed based on child disability.
Brigance Diagnostic Inventory of Early Development–II (Brigance, 2004)	Evaluation for eligibility and program intervention: criterion- and norm-referenced	0–7 years	Widely used due to ease of developing IFSP and IEP objectives.
Carolina Curriculum for Infants and Toddlers with Special Needs, Third Edition (Johnson-Martin et al., 2004) and Carolina Curriculum for Preschoolers with Special Needs, Second Edition (Johnson-Martin, et al., 2004)	Curriculum-based assessment: program intervention	0–24 months 24 months–5 years	Time consuming and difficult to locate items in protocol
Denver II (Frankenburg, et. al., 1992)	Screening: standardized, norm-referenced	0–6 years	Quick administration, clear procedures, materials provided in compact kit
The Early Intervention Developmental Profile (Rogers, Donovan, D'Eugenio, et al.)	Evaluation for eligibility and program intervention: criterion-referenced with corresponding age ranges	0–3 years	Items are clearly explained, but inexperienced examiner must refer to manual for administration

continued

Table 5.1. Assessment Instruments for Young Children–*Continued.*

Instruments	Purpose/type of instrument	Age Range	Feasibility
Hawaii Early Learning Profile (HELP Checklist) (Furuno et.al., 2005)	Programing intervention: criterion-referenced with corresponding age ranges	0–3 years	Items clearly explained, but inexperienced examiner must refer to manual for administration
HELP for Preschoolers Checklist (VORT Corp, 1995)	Program intervention: criterion-referenced with age ranges	3–6 years	Clear definitions: difficult to assess play skills
HELP Strands (adaptation of original HELP) (Parks, 2004)	Program intervention: curriculum-based, developmental assessment	0–3 years	Descriptive definitions on strand scoring protocol: procedures for scoring clearly delineated
Movement Assessment of Infants (MAI) (Chandler, et. al., 1980)	Program intervention: criterion-referenced	0–12 months	Timely to administer, lacks organization, but quantifies quality of infant movement
Peabody Developmental Motor Scales (Folio & Fewell, 2000)	Gross and fine motor assessment for eligibility and program planning: standardized, norm-referenced	0–83 months	Comprehensive, time consuming
Preschool Developmental Profile (D'Eugenio & Moersch, 1981)	Evaluation for eligibility and program intervention: criterion-referenced with corresponding age ranges	3–5 years	Items are clearly explained in manual
Transdisciplinary Play-Based Assessment (TPBA), (Linder, 1993)	Functional approach to assessment of young children evaluated in six phases during natural play interactions	6 months–6 years	Thorough evaluation of all domains in friendly natural play setting: no normative data, no reflex assessment, nor explanation of equilibrium responses. Time and scheduling constraints may cause difficulty in evaluation.

ASSESSMENT INSTRUMENTS

Screening Instruments

Screening infants' or toddlers' motor abilities is often completed by medical personnel. Screening for preschoolers who exhibit motor difficulties is frequently completed informally by various educational professionals. Because movement specialists infrequently screen young children, only three instruments are described in this category.

Ages and Stages Questionnaire: A Parent-Completed, Child-Monitoring System, Second Edition (ASQ)

The ASQ (Bricker, Squires, Mounts, Potter, Nickel, Twombly, & Farrell, 1999) is a screening instrument for young children ages 4 months–5 years that is used to identify a child at risk for developmental delay and to monitor a child's developmental progress. The instrument includes 19 levels at 2-month increments up to the age of 24 months, 3-month increments up to 36 months, and 6-month increments up to age 5 years. Each leveled questionnaire contains 30 items that can be administered in 10–20 minutes by parents, teachers, social workers, or medical or mental health providers. Questions are presented to indicate whether a behavior is present, sometimes present, or not yet apparent. Responses are converted to point values and then compared to a cut-off score. Each level provides scores in communication, gross motor, fine motor, problem solving, and personal-social domains.

Critique

The ASQ is a screening instrument that indicates whether a child needs further evaluation. It is low cost, easy and quick to administer, and has Spanish, French, and Korean translations. The 4th to 6th-grade reading level for the questionnaire and items that include simple illustrations permit adults with varying educational levels to administer the questionnaire. Technical data are provided in the technical report section of the user's guide. There are limited data concerning the normative sample of 2,008 children and although the represented samples of Caucasians and African Americans are acceptable, Native Americans are overrepresented and Latino/Hispanic families are underrepresented. Test-retest reliability exceeds 90 percent agreement, inter-rater reliability is high, and correlation with other assessment instruments is also high (.83). Validity is considered moderate. Additionally, at some of the age levels, there is a high rate of false positives and false negatives. The test developers state that this is due to the range of socioeconomic status and educational levels of the questionnaire respondents and that this rate is adequate because the instrument is used as a "first-level" system for screening.

Battelle Developmental Inventory Screening Test

The Battelle Developmental Inventory Screening Test (Newborg, 2004) is one section provided in the Battelle Developmental Inventory, Second Edition (BDI-2). The screening test is a standardized norm-referenced instrument for children from birth through eight years of age and covers five domains: (a) personal or social, (b) adaptive, (c) motor, (d) communication, and (e) cognition. The items are a subset of items from the full BDI-2 that can be scored by structured testing, observation, or interview. General adaptations are provided for individuals with motor impairments, visual impairments, hearing impairments, or emotional disabilities (see Figure 5.7). Cutoff scores are provided to determine the children that may need additional assessment.

Critique

Within the motor domain, the subdomains of fine motor, perceptual motor, and gross motor are included; however, the number of items is very limited. The age increments are large and the limited number of gross motor and fine motor abilities provides minimal information that would be applicable to most movement specialists. Advantages of this instrument include: (a) most professionals can administer this assessment, (b) it can be completed quickly (entire screening in 10–30 minutes), (c) caregivers can be present during the testing, and (d) informal observations can be used to score test items.

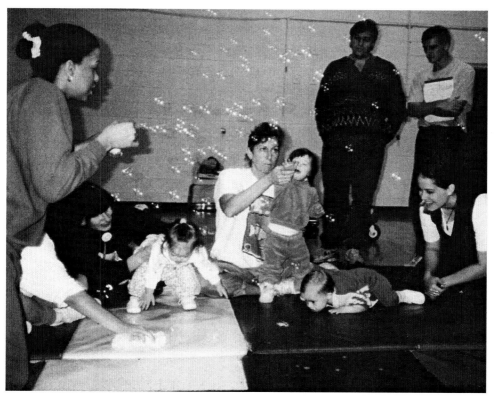

Figure 5.7. An evaluator observes and assesses motor development skills of several young children during play interactions with their families. The Battelle Developmental Screening Test permits scoring through observations.

Denver II

The Denver II (Frankenburg, Dodds, Archer, Bresnick, Maschka, Edelman, & Shapiro, 1992) is a widely-used standardized screening instrument. It is a norm-referenced measure of four developmental areas: (a) personal-social, (b) fine motor-adaptive, (c) language, and (d) gross motor (see Figure 5.8). Evaluation of test behavior has been added to the most recent revision and includes a rating of the child's attention span, compliance, interest in surroundings, and fearfulness. The Denver II is designed for use in a clinical setting by trained professionals and paraprofessionals to provide a description of a child 0–6 years of age who may be "at-risk" for developmental delay. The Denver II includes 125 items and can be administered in approximately 20 minutes. It provides specific criteria for determining

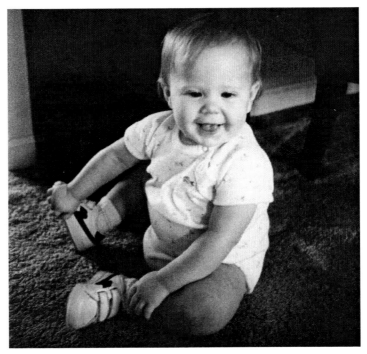

Figure 5.8. Sitting independently is a developmental skill routinely assessed in a screening instrument such as the Denver II.

whether the results of a screening are normal, suspect, unstable, or indicate need for referral. The Denver II training manual should be referred to when calculating the child's age. Drawing of the age line is critical in interpretation of this assessment instrument. The test allows for adjustment of prematurity for children born more than two weeks prior to the expected delivery date until the child is two years of age.

Critique

The Denver II is recognized throughout the pediatric medical profession as a highly reliable measure of child development. It is often used in health clinics for routine screening at periodic intervals. Data from the clinics are often the basis of a referral for a more thorough evaluation. The administration instructions and procedures are clearly delineated in the manual and the protocol is neatly placed on one sheet. Materials required for administration are provided in a small, compact kit. Adjustments in scoring for a premature child allow for a more valid prediction of developmental delay and referral for further testing. Although the items on the gross motor and fine motor-adaptive sections are adequate for screening, there is no reference to muscle tone or reflex analysis throughout the test nor is there adequate assessment of hand function.

Eligibility Instruments

Child eligibility for special education services must be determined according to state or federal guidelines. Various standardized and criterion-referenced tests are utilized for this purpose and therefore are described below.

Battelle Developmental Inventory, Second Edition

The Battelle Developmental Inventory (BDI-2) (Newborg, 2004) is used to identify children with disabilities who are eligible for services, to plan and provide intervention services, and to analyze functional capabilities of children ages 0–7.11 years. It is a comprehensive, standardized, norm-referenced assessment battery, with 341 items grouped in five domains: (a) personal-social, (b) adaptive, (c) motor, (d) communication, and (e) cognitive. It is recommended that the test administrator study the manuals and practice administration prior to administering the instrument to individuals with disabilities. Each item can be scored by structured administration, observation, or interview; it is recommended that the examiner use the method that will provide the best data. Technical data for this assessment are provided in the manual. High reliability is demonstrated for subdomain, domain, and full-test composite levels. Concurrent and criterion related validity is established on the original BDI and other acceptable assessment instruments. A curriculum linked to the BDI is available. It provides instructional activities for program planning in each of the five domains plus activities for caregivers and special events.

The motor domain items are grouped into three subdomains: fine motor, perceptual motor, and gross motor (see Figure 5.9). Most subdomains are divided into 5-month increments (although some age ranges span 1 year) with the number of items in each subdomain increment ranging from 1–5.

Critique

The BDI-2 is popular for use in programs serving young children with disabilities and the movement specialist is often one of the transdisciplinary team members involved in administering this assessment in arena style. Several new features are included in this updated version of the BDI: expanded range of items in all domains, colorful items and child-friendly manipulatives, scripted Interview items with follow-up probes that provide complete information on the child's development, updated comprehensive norms based on 2,500 children, and web-based scoring.

However, this instrument is time-consuming, taking 1–2 hours to administer. At certain specified ages, there are an insufficient number of items to make clear decisions concerning the child's motor abilities. This lessens the usefulness of the subdomains in program planning.

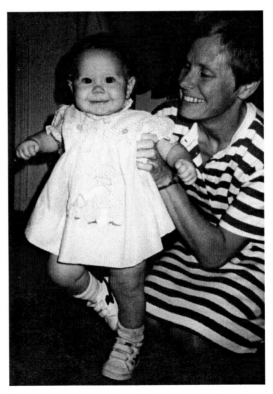

Figure 5.9. The mother provides support while assessing the skill of "making stepping movements in place with support," which usually occurs between 8–10 months of age.

Also, within some specific age increments, skills are assessed in different subdomains. This requires the examiner to "jump around" in the test booklet to adequately assess all motor development items at that specific age.

The Bayley Scales of Infant and Toddler Development, Third Edition

The Bayley Scales of Infant and Toddler Development, Third Edition (Bayley III) (Bayley, 2006) is a standardized, norm-referenced instrument that assesses infants and young children between the ages of 1 month and 42 months. Its major purpose is to determine developmental delay and to provide information to guide intervention; however, it is also used to indicate progress, to provide information to caregivers, and for research. The most recent edition identifies an individual's strengths, abilities, competencies, and deficits across 5 domains: cognition, language, motor, adaptive behavior, and social-emotional. There is also a Behavior Observation Inventory (a sixth scale) that is completed by the caregiver and examiner to provide further information about the child's behavior at home and in the testing environment. All materials required for testing are provided in a compact rolling kit. There are specific qualifications for purchasing this instrument and detailed training and rehearsal are needed prior to test administration; however, motor development specialists have the knowledge and abilities to utilize the motor scale.

Specific procedures must be followed during administration of the Cognition, Language, and Motor scales of the Bayley-III, while completion of the Social-Emotional and Adaptive Behavior Scales are completed by the parent or primary caregiver in questionnaire format. Directions are easy to follow and test item administration occurs within child-like activities. Test administration takes approximately 50 minutes for infants under age 12 months and 90 minutes for older preschool children. Each item is scored after the stimuli or testing materials are presented by the examiner and credit is awarded if the child successfully performs the task. Items can also be scored as correct if they are observed incidentally at another time during testing. Caregivers may be involved in administration of some items and input may be provided for a task, but the child is not given credit for passing unless the examiner has observed successful completion of the item.

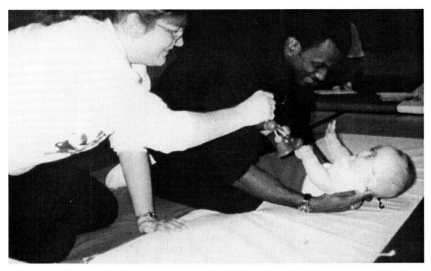

Figure 5.10. As infant development proceeds, lifting head while supported at the shoulders is a skill that is often assessed (e.g., Bayley-III, 20006).

Accommodations for a child's disability are allowed when comparing the child's performance to normative data; however, modifications are not permitted. An accommodation is a change in the way the test is administered (either how the test is presented or a variation in how the child responds), while a modification is a change in content of the test. There are specific accommodation features embedded within the Bayley-III that were developed for statewide assessments. The examiner must use caution when interpreting test scores of a child with disabilities when other individualized, nonstandardized accommodations have been made.

Psychometric data are provided in the Bayley III manual (2006). The sample of 1,700 children included 10 percent children with specific clinical diagnoses (e.g., Down Syndrome, Cerebral Palsy, Pervasive Developmental Disorder, premature birth, language impairment), and was stratified on key demographic variables, including geographic location, age, sex, and parent education level. Normative data are provided in 10-day increments from 16 days of age to 5 months 15 days, and in monthly intervals for other aged children. The overall average reliability coefficients for the subtests range from .91 to .86. Validity was found to be acceptable based on test content, internal structure, and relation to other measures (e.g., Bayley Scales of Infant

Development-II, WPPSI-III). Additionally, the Bayley-III was found to be valid for children with specific clinical diagnoses (e.g., Down syndrome, Pervasive Development Disorder, Cerebral Palsy, Specific Language Impairment). Empirical support was therefore provided for utilizing this instrument to differentiate between children who are typical and children with diagnosed clinical impairments.

The Motor Scale of the Bayley-III includes 138 items which assess gross and fine motor control (see Figure 5.10). The gross motor section (72 items) includes movements associated with head control and isolated limb movements, trunk control, rolling, crawling and creeping, sitting, standing, walking, running, jumping and balance; while the fine motor section (66 items) involves eye movements, grasping, prehension, adaptive use of writing instruments, imitation of hand movements and paper-pencil tasks, and cutting. There are also items which assess the areas of sensory integration, perceptual-motor integration, motor planning, and play.

Critique

The Bayley-III has been expanded in its newest edition and provides a thorough assessment of children age birth through 42 months. The number of items has been expanded and allows for easier identification of lower functioning infants and higher functioning toddlers. The number of fine and gross motor skill items has increased and provides a thorough assessment of the motor domain. Components of play and perceptual-motor integration are also evaluated, but within the cognitive domain. The administration manual of this instrument is clearly written, and provides an unambiguous description of items and scoring procedures. Some pictures are provided. Items for testing are provided and come in a compact carry-case. However, for some of the gross motor items, other equipment must either by available on-site, or diagrams are provided for construction. In this third edition, the norms have been updated and include children with a wider array of disabilities. Also, caregiver input is allowed and play-like administration is possible. The Bayley-III does not assess primitive reflexes, equilibrium responses, and muscle tone, which are all important components when analyzing movement abilities and difficulties of individuals with disabilities. Also, the age range is restrictive and is not applicable to all preschool-aged children.

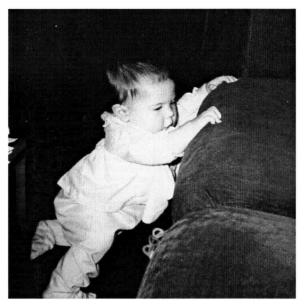

Figure 5-11. The ability to pull to stand via half-kneel reflects an acquisition of total body strength as well as coordination.

Brigance Diagnostic Inventory of Early Development-II

The Brigance Diagnostic Inventory of Early Development-II (IED-II) (Brigance, 2004) is a criterion-referenced and norm-referenced instrument for children from birth to seven years of age. It includes skill sequences that assess the following areas: (a) psychomotor, (b) self-help, (c) speech and language, (d) general knowledge and comprehension, and (e) early academic skills. When a child has difficulty within the skill sequences, the examiner can more specifically analyze performance through utilization of comprehensive skill sequences. Within the psychomotor domain, the preambulatory section includes four skills sequences, the gross motor skills section includes 10 skill sequences, and the fine motor section includes five skill sequences. Within the comprehensive preambulatory motor skill and behaviors section, 53 supine behaviors, 21 prone behaviors, 25 sitting behaviors, and 33 standing behaviors are assessed. The skill sequences include items to be observed in each of the positions, for example, reflexes, visual control, head control, gross motor, fine motor, and hand function. Included in the suggested assessment procedures are relevant informational notes providing beneficial descriptions of muscle tone and primitive/protective reflexes of the newborn child. Comprehensive skills within the gross motor domain include 19 standing skills, 25 walking skills, 20 stairs and climbing skills, 17 running skills, 29 jumping skills, 12 balance beam skills and 15 rolling and throwing skills. The comprehensive fine motor section includes 18 general eye/finger/hand manipulative skills, 26 block tower building skills, 21 prehandwriting skills, 18 form skills, and 16 cutting skills. This section also includes supplemental skills with puzzles, brush painting, and clay (see Figure 5.11).

Caregiver interview, observation by the examiner during unstructured play, games, or class or group activities, and examiner administration of the test items with alterations (demonstration) as needed, may be used to score the items. No specific qualifications are required for test administration. Pictures and explanations enable easy administration of the items (see Figure 5.12). There are intricate skills listed with accompanying pictures and descriptive details to assist the examiner in scoring the protocol.

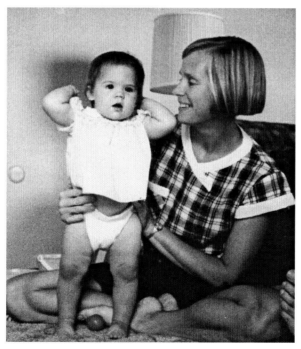

Figure 5.12. Supporting one's weight while standing with assistance is a precursor to independent standing.

Critique

The assessment begins with the child in supine position to facilitate eye contact between the child and the examiner and to allow for easy assessment of vertical and horizontal eye movements. The positioning sequences and detailed informational notes and pictures in this pre-ambulatory section provide an excellent assessment format for the novice examiner. For individuals who are less familiar with aspects of very early childhood development, this assessment instrument provides clear information to assist in determining skill levels.

Skills within the gross and fine motor sequences are also clearly defined and criteria for acceptable performance and discontinue rules are provided. However, it is difficult to determine the child's specific developmental age level within a particular skill sequence, and the examiner arbitrarily decides at what level the child is performing. The

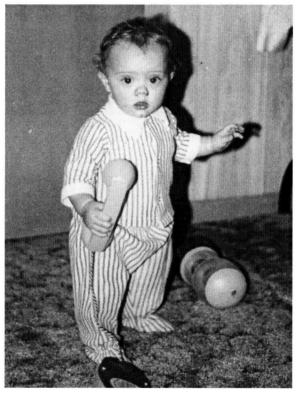

Figure 5.13. When an infant first learns to stand without support, she may demonstrate a wide base of support with arms flexed and raised to maintain balance.

age ranges are very wide and skills are not always identified by specific years and months. However, because of the normative data and the usefulness for developing IFSP or IEP objectives, this instrument is widely used.

Developmental Programming for Infants and Young Children (Rogers & Donovan, 1981)

Developmental Programming for Infants and Young Children consists of **Early Intervention Developmental Profile (EIDP)** (Rogers & Donovan, 1981) and **the Preschool Developmental Profile** (D'Eugenio & Moersch, 1981). Both profiles assess six developmental areas for children: (a) perceptual or fine motor, (b) cognition, (c) language, (d) social or emotional, (e) self-care, and (f) gross motor. These criterion-referenced assessment instruments provide age ranges corresponding to the development of specific skills. The development of both instruments is based on the Piagetian Theory of sensorimotor intelligence. Descriptions for administering each item and the scoring process which identifies ceiling and basal levels utilizing a pass or fail criteria are included. Materials needed for administration are listed in the manual but must be obtained and organized by the examiner. General alterations for instrument administration are provided in the manual but are not specific for each item.

The EIDP includes 77 items in the gross motor scale and 48 items in the fine motor or perceptual scale developmentally sequenced in 2–4 month increments (see Figure 5.13). The PDP has 35 perceptual or fine motor items and 57 gross motor items developmentally sequenced in 6-month increments. A curriculum of stimulation activities for items up through age 35 months is provided when an individual fails respective items. The perceptual or fine motor score suggests the beginning age range for administration of the remaining scales.

Critique

The EIDP has been a widely-used instrument for young children during past decades. The test manuals provide instructions for administration, scoring, and interpretation that are clear and easy to understand. However, when the examiner is not experienced with the items it requires that he or she refer to the appropriate manual for test item descriptions.

Of the instruments which assess several developmental domains, the EIDP includes the most comprehensive assessment of primitive reflexes and equilibrium reactions. Excellent pictorial diagrams are provided in the manual to assist with intervention activities for young children.

Peabody Developmental Motor Scales, Second Edition

Peabody Developmental Motor Scales, Second Edition (PDMS-2) (Folio & Fewell, 2000) evaluates gross and fine motor development of children ages 0 to 72 months. With the set of remediation activities, it can also be used to monitor a child's development through repeated measures. The PDMS-2 is a standardized norm-referenced instrument with a corresponding motor activity program manual to direct program planning. The gross motor section includes 170 items in the areas of reflexes (8 items), stationary measures (30 items), locomotion (89 items), and object manipulation (24 items). The fine motor section includes 98 items in the areas of reaching and grasping (26 items), and visual motor integration (72 items) (see Figure 5.14). All items are directly tested and credit is not given for report from caregiver or teacher.

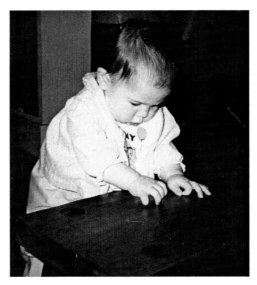

Figure 5.14. This child demonstrates the more general skill of standing and is practicing the more specific skills of palmar and pincer grasp.

Critique

The Peabody Developmental Motor Scales (second edition) is a comprehensive test of motor development for young children which also provides intervention activities. It can be administered quite quickly, in 20–30 minutes, and the criteria for scoring are objective and explicit. Special training is not required. Scores can be compiled manually or through the use of a computer program. Profile/summary forms allow the examiner to graphically display a child's performance that is useful to clarify the child's performance to family members. Norms were developed from 2,003 children from British Columbia, Canada and throughout the United States. Acceptable age ranges, geographical diversity, gender and racial diversity were carefully controlled. The assessment provides standard scores (percentile, motor age, and developmental motor quotient) to make determinations about eligibility for motor services within special education. Validity and reliability are acceptable, but it should be noted that the standardization sample included small numbers of children with disabilities. Additionally it should be noted that many of the testing items are not included in the testing kit.

Instruments for Program Planning

Assessment, Evaluation, and Programming System for Infants and Children, Second Edition (AEPS)

The AEPS is a comprehensive system that coordinates assessment, goal development, intervention, and ongoing monitoring. The testing leads to the development of goals which link directly to intervention content and procedures. The primary purpose of the system is to assist professionals and families in identifying and monitoring developmentally appropriate educational targets and in planning individualized intervention. Instructions are provided for both center and home-based settings, and the family is an important component in the entire assessment and intervention process.

The AEPS is composed of 4 volumes: the Administration Guide (Bricker, Pretti-Frontczak, Johnson, & Straka, 2002), the Test (Bricker, Capt, Pretti-Frontczak, & Johnson, 2002), Curriculum for Birth to Three Years (Bricker & Waddell, 2002), and Curriculum for Three to Six Years (Bricker & Waddell, 2002). The Administration Guide presents information on the conceptual and organizational structure and an explanation of the system, the interpretation of the testing, family involvement in the testing, and team collaboration. The AEPS Test contains test items for both Birth to Three Years and Three to Six Years, and includes skills in six domains: (a) fine motor, (b) gross motor, (c) adaptive, (d) cognitive, (e) social-communication, and (f) social. Volumes 3 and 4 include curriculum activities and intervention strategies in each of the domains for children birth to three and three to six years. Environmental arrangements and modifications are also provided. Adjunct materials to monitor child progress and assist in working with families are included in the AEPS. A family report of child abilities and an assessment of family interests are included. The assessment instruments for each level are criterion-referenced and curriculum-based and assess functional skills of children who are at risk or who are disabled. Each domain is divided into strands which contain a series of test items (goals and objectives) in hierarchical, sequential order from earliest attained (easiest) to skills which are attained at older ages (more difficult) (see Figure 5.15). The test objectives represent discrete skills which pinpoint a child's level within the specific skill sequence. It is suggested that test goals and objectives can be used for IEP or IFSP annual goals and quarterly objectives. Developmental age norms are not provided because the authors of the AEPS consider the comparison of performance to age norms as questionable value in program planning.

The intended users of this system include interventionists (teachers) and allied health professionals. Although observation during play, planned activities, and/or regular routines is preferred, assessment information can be collected by direct testing or through reports from parents, caregivers, therapists, the examiner, or written documentation (e.g., medical reports). Specific criteria for scoring observations or direct testing is provided in the test protocol and scored as either 2 = consistently meets criterion, 1 = inconsistently meets criterion, and 0 = does not meet criterion. Modifications for disability groups are included. Seven activity plans to facilitate a testing environment are provided in the manual. The authors suggest that testing occur over several days.

The AEPS links assessment data to the development of the IFSP or IEP. The AEPS Curriculum, Birth to Three and Three to Six Years (Bricker & Waddell, 2002) present the theory of activity-based inter-

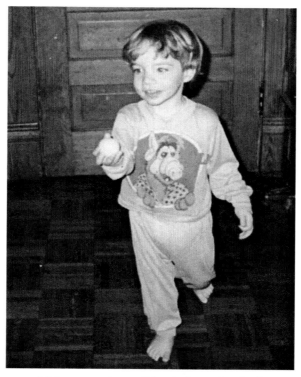

Figure 5.15. As young children practice walking independently they acquire a reciprocal pattern displayed by cross-lateral use of the arms and legs. This child is exhibiting a less mature, homo-lateral walking position

vention that incorporates the assessment and intervention processes into the child's daily activities and life experiences. Activity-based intervention enables multiple targeted objectives to be addressed in a single activity that a child typically engages in due to his or her interests. The AEPS provides activities for each domain. Goals and objectives as well as teaching and environmental considerations are included. For children from three to six years, the curriculum provides general intervention considerations and suggested activities to address individual learning styles, rather than addressing specific instructional sequences.

AEPS Birth to Three includes developmental skills from 1 month to 3 years, but is generally appropriate for children with disabilities 1 month to 6 years of age. In the gross motor domain there are four strands, including: (a) movement and locomotion in supine and prone positions, (b) balance in sitting, (c) balance and mobility in standing, walking, running and stair walking, and (d) play skills. The two fine motor strands include (a) reach, grasp and release, and (b) functional use of fine motor skills. For the birth to three year range, there are 26 items including objectives and goals in the two strands of the fine motor domain and 55 items (goals and objectives) in the four strands of the gross motor domain. This level of the AEPS is generally appropriate for children with disabilities with chronological ages ranging from 3 to 8 years. Within the three-to-six-year range, the fine motor domain is divided into the following strands: (a) bilateral motor coordination, with 5 items including goals and objectives; and (b) emergent writing, with 10 items (goals and objectives) (total of 15 items). The gross motor domain is divided into the following two strands: (a) balance and mobility in standing, walking, running, and stair walking (4 items including objectives and goals); and (b) play skills (13 items including goals and objectives).

Critique

This assessment system has been designed for the classroom environment, and would be useful for a movement specialist if he or she completes the assessment with other early intervention professionals. The system links assessment and intervention and is very useful for programming. The system values caregiver input and allows caregiver observations to be used as valid test data. It also surveys caregiver interests. The curriculum associated with the AEPS assessment is very convenient and useful for teachers. Concurrent goals and objectives listed from other strands can be incorporated into each planned activity.

Items on both levels of this assessment in the two motor domains are extremely limited. Although the AEPS is considered appropriate for individuals with severe disabilities, inhibition of primitive reflexes and development of equilibrium reactions are not included for children birth to three years. These are important to the movement interventionist when designing functional gross motor tasks to facilitate successful movement of infants, toddlers, and preschoolers throughout the environment. There are also "gaps" in the motor sequences involving the development of head and trunk control in prone and supine. Additionally, play skills in the motor section begin with high level skills (i.e., jumping down and jumping forward) which may be inappropriate for young children with developmental delays. Some related manipulation and play tasks can be found in the strands titled "Causality," "Imitation" and "Interaction with objects" (Cognitive Domain); however, this organization makes summarization of play abilities within the context of gross and fine motor abilities very confusing for the motor evaluator.

Carolina Curriculum for Infants and Toddlers with Special Needs (Third Edition) (CCI) (Johnson-Martin, Jens, Attermeier, & Hacker, 2004)

Carolina Curriculum for Preschoolers with Special Needs (Second Edition) (CCPSN) (Johnson-Martin, Jens, Attermeier, Hacker, 2004)

The Carolina Curriculum includes two volumes: The Carolina Curriculum for Infants and Toddlers with Special Needs (CCITSN), (third edition) and the Carolina Curriculum for Preschoolers with Special Needs (CCPSN) (second edition). The Carolina Curriculum system includes curriculum-based instruments linking to extensive and thorough programs for intervention. The CCITSN is designed for young children between the ages of birth to 24 months and The CCPSN accommodates children beyond the 24-month level up to 5 years of age who have mild to severe disabilities. Both assessments are organized according to skill areas with a curriculum sequence that provides developmental age ranges for each skill. The Carolina Curriculum is a criterion referenced system that professionals can use in home-, school- or center-based environments with other teachers, family members and other service providers. The system includes an assessment log and developmental progress charts.

The CCITSN instrument includes 24 specific skill sequences in the five developmental domains of cognition, communication, social adaptation, fine motor, and gross motor. There is an emphasis on sensorimotor development (e.g., visual pursuit, object permanence, auditory localization, attention and memory, visual perception). Curriculum sequences not traditionally included as a part of assessment instruments are: (a) visual pursuit and object permanence, (b) auditory localization and object permanence, (c) understanding space, and (d) tactile integration. These sequences are based on several classic models of sensorimotor development (Bly, 1980; Bobath, 1948; Pikler, 1971; Rood, 1954). Assessment of gross and fine motor skills are organized

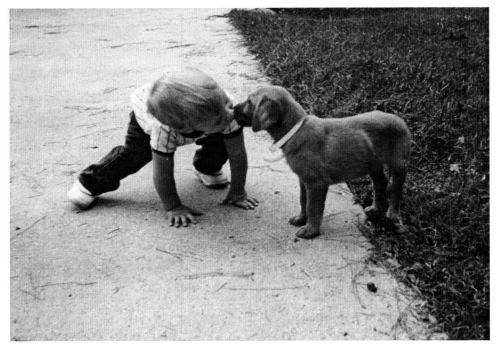

Figure 5.16. This young child demonstrates the ability to squat (or stoop) during play, a skill assessed on the Carolina Curriculum for Infants and Toddlers with Special Needs.

within skill sequences: items on play are limited to functional use of play objects and symbolic play in the cognitive domain and several interactive play items in the social domain. Although the instrument was field-tested nationally, validity and reliability data were not included for the curriculum-based assessment.

Items on the CCPSN were developed from clinical experience of the authors, the research literature, and a variety of published assessment instruments. The fine motor domain includes strands in the areas of motor imitation, grasp and manipulation, bilateral skills, tool use, and visual motor skills. The gross motor domain includes strands delineating upright posture and locomotion, upright balance, and upright ball play, and upright outdoor play (see Figure 5.16). Symbolic play skills are included in the cognition domain.

Critique

The CCITSN and CCPSN are each considered one of the better

curriculum-based instruments for their respective age groups. Although the authors designed the curricula to be used with children who have mild to severe disabilities, the variability of the curriculum sequences (e.g., visual pursuit and object permanence, auditory localization, understanding space, functional use of objects, and symbolic play) and details for teaching self-help and fine motor skills provide excellent activities for children with physical disabilities. Due to the comprehensiveness of the curricula, both instruments are time-consuming to administer and the equipment requirements are extensive. It is also time-consuming for the movement specialist to assemble items within the protocols that one might select for assessing skills in the protocols, although many items are typically found in the classroom. However, the CCITSN and CCPSN are very useful for the early interventionist in the classroom environment when identifying programmatic skills. The instruments provide adaptations for various exceptionalities and suggestions for use in daily routines.

The Hawaii Early Learning Profile (HELP) Curriculum and Assessment Materials

The HELP Curriculum and Assessment Materials include *Inside HELP, Administration and Reference Manual for the Hawaii Early Learning Profile* (Parks, 2006), *HELP Strands* (Parks, 2004); *HELP Checklist: Ages Birth to Three Years* (Furuno, O'Reilly, Hosaka, Inatsuka, Zeisloft-Falvey, & Ailman, 1988); *HELP Charts and HELP Activity Guide* (Furuno, O'Reilly, Hosaka, Inatsuka, Ailman, & Zeisloft, 2005); *HELP at Home* (Parks, Furuno, O'Reilly, Inatsuka, Hosaka, & Zeisloft-Falbey, 1995); and *HELP When the Parent has Disabilities* (Parks, 1999).

The Hawaii Early Learning Profile is a comprehensive system of assessment and programming for children ages birth to 36 months. The purposes or objectives of each HELP component are somewhat different. The HELP Checklist and HELP Strands are the main assessment components. *Help for Preschoolers, Assessment Checklist: Ages 3–6* (VORT, 1995) was developed as an extension of HELP Birth to 3 and follows the format of the original HELP Checklist. The original HELP materials included 685 developmental skills or behaviors in a checklist (HELP Checklist) and chart (HELP Chart) format that were reviewed by programs in 35 states and 7 different countries. Both the chart and checklist are organized according to age ranges within six

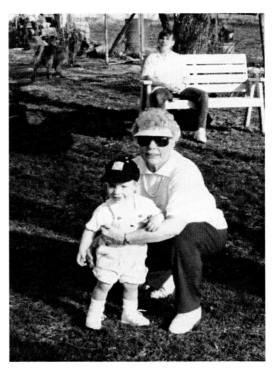

Figure 5.17. "Stands, holding on" is an item on the HELP Checklist and Strands.

developmental domains: (a) cognitive, (b) language, (c) gross motor, (d) fine motor, (e) social-emotional, and (f) self-help.

The HELP for Preschoolers Checklist: Ages 3– 6 (VORT, 1995) includes 5 areas of motor development and provides associated curricular activities for each item. Eighty-seven skills are assessed in the gross motor area and 38 skills are assessed in the fine motor area. Play skills are evaluated in 14 of 22 interpersonal relations skills. There is also HELP for Preschoolers Assessment Standards (VORT, 2004) and HELP for Preschoolers Assessment and Curriculum Guide (VORT, 1999) which present similar information in different formats.

The HELP Strands (Parks, 2004) is a curriculum-based developmental assessment adapted from the original HELP Checklist and Chart. It was field-tested over a 3-year period with more than 200 infants and toddlers to determine the adequacy of the hierarchical sequencing of skills within strands. Each strand focuses on specific hierarchical skills within an identified key concept. For example, within the key concept or strand "weight-bearing in standing, the skill of "stands, holding on" is one of seven skills assessed (see Figure 5.17). The gross motor domain of the HELP Strands includes 83 assessment items in 7 strands for ages 0–15 months, and 69 items in 8 strands for ages 15–36 months. The fine motor domain includes 104 items in seven strands. Descriptive definitions are provided on the Strands form for each skill. For example, "stands holding on–several seconds at chest high support; hands only for balance; not leaning." Play items are placed in one section, "Social Interactions and Play."

Critique

The HELP Strands includes more assessment items in the gross motor and fine motor areas than most other instruments and also has more items within smaller age ranges (see Figure 5.18). The procedures for scoring are clearly delineated in the HELP Strands, which is especially useful for students, teachers, or caregivers who are unfamiliar with developmental progressions of very young children. The organization of the skills within the HELP Strands allows for an easy transition from one skill to another, thus facilitating administration (see Figure 5.19).

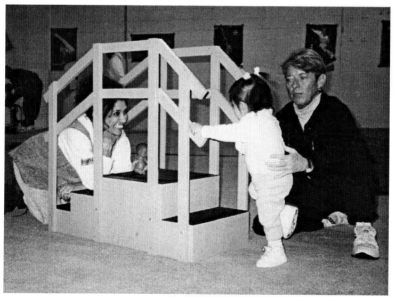

Figure 5.18. The ability to walk upstairs holding the rail usually emerges between 15–18 months of age.

This lessens the physical demands on the young child and the examiner which ultimately increases reliability of the assessment. Fox example, if the child had to complete activities in prone, supine and then again in prone, the child would become very tired from changing to each position. This format of administration also reduces the stimulation of primitive reflexes. Within the HELP Strands, play items are conveniently placed in one section "Social Interactions and Play," which also facilitates using this assessment by caregivers and inexperienced teachers.

Movement Assessment of Infants (MAI)

The Movement Assessment of Infants (MAI) (Chandler, Andrews, & Swanson, 1980) assesses the quality of an infant's motor development from birth to age 12 months. It is a criterion-referenced assessment that evaluates the areas of muscle tone, primitive reflexes, automatic reactions, and volitional movement. Other developmental domains are not included in this assessment. The instrument includes six items in muscle tone, 11 primitive reflexes, 14 automatic reactions, and 23 volitional movements, and further includes an asymmetry

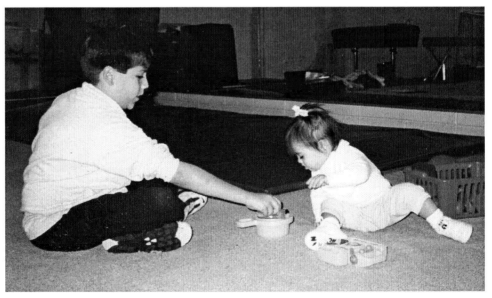

Figure 5.19. Pivoting in sitting and twisting the truck to reach across midline for play objects is an item on the HELP Strands.

index and summary items in each section. "The strength of the MAI lies in its quantification of quality of infant movement" (Einarsson-Backes, & Stewart, 1992, p. 226).

The MAI is intended to be administered by medically-trained personnel, or "others who have specialized knowledge and experience in infant development" (Chandler et al., 1980, p. 13). The adapted physical educator would most typically administer this instrument with physical or occupational therapists in a team setting. Brief explanations of each item are provided; however, specificity is limited and it is necessary that the examiner have prior knowledge of assessing reflexes and movement positions for young infants. The sections on muscle tone and primitive reflexes include good descriptive information for determining movement deficits. The section on volitional movement enables the examiner to complete extensive multisensory (visual, auditory, vestibular, tactile) analysis that is useful for educational programming.

Critique

The MAI is timely to administer and does not provide normative data that is required for determining eligibility for service delivery. The scoring criteria and the scoring protocol are poorly organized making continuity of administration difficult. For the adapted physical educator this instrument is recommended for use as a resource rather than an instrument to be administered in its entirety.

Transdisciplinary Play-Based Assessment

Transdisciplinary Play-Based Assessment (TPBA) (Linder, 1993) is a functional approach to assessment of young children age 6 months to 6 years with the primary purpose to impact the intervention process. The domains of cognitive, language and communication, sensorimotor, and social-emotional development are assessed by team members in a play environment. Caregivers, appropriate educational personnel and medical professionals comprise the team. The assessment occurs with a play facilitator, caregiver(s), and a peer in approximately 60 to 90 minutes. Prior to the assessment, a planning meeting is held to discuss activities, materials, the environment for the play session, the structure of the session, and assignment of team members' roles.

The format of the assessment involves six phases. During each

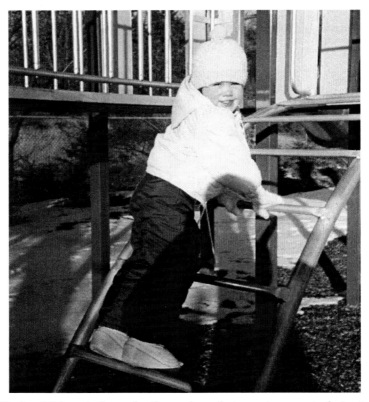

Figure 5.20. As children independently explore their environment, their strength and coordination continue to develop and they begin to demonstrate bilateral movements of the head, trunk, and extremities.

phase, team members observe the child and seek to answer questions suggested in the assessment protocol that are pertinent to the child's developmental status. Each phase serves a specific purpose for evaluation. **Unstructured facilitation** is phase I. The play facilitator follows the child's lead in any play activity, imitates behavior or vocalizations, engages in conversation, and interacts in parallel, associative, or cooperative play (see Figure 5.20).

During **structured facilitation**, phase II, the facilitator requests the child to perform specific cognitive or language tasks that were not observed during phase I. In the third phase, child interaction, a peer is introduced to the play setting to enable professionals to observe interaction behaviors. During the fourth phase, **parent-child interaction**, parents (or caregivers) engage in play activities with their child

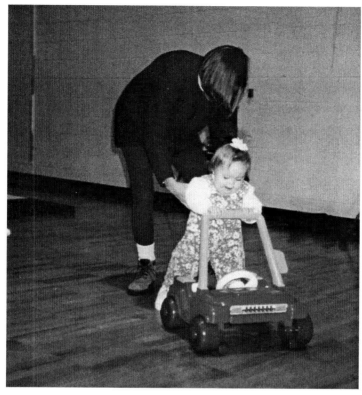

Figure 5.21. The play facilitator provides support and encouragement for walking during phase V (motor play) of the Transdisciplinary Play-Based Assessment.

that they typically engage in at home. **Motor play** (phase V) involves a structured and unstructured component (see Figure 5.21). During unstructured motor play, the play facilitator follows, encourages, and initiates motor play on various types of equipment. A motor professional (e.g., adapted physical educator, occupational therapist, physical therapist) may also involve the child in more structured activities and hands-on activities. The final phase (VI) of the assessment, snack, allows observation of social interactions, adaptive behavior, self-help skills, and oral motor development.

Sensorimotor development is evaluated during the motor play phase of the assessment. The child's ability to accomplish motor milestones and the quality of the child's performance is determined. Observation guidelines are provided in question format for the observer to determine the child's abilities in eight areas: (a) general

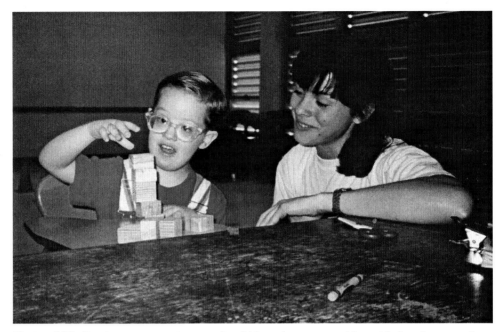

Figure 5.22. During assessment, care should be taken to provide guided assistance when presenting an unfamiliar task to a child.

appearance of movement; (b) muscle tone, strength, and endurance; (c) reactivity to sensory input; (d) stationary positions used for play; (e) mobility in play; (f) other developmental achievements (e.g., jumping, climbing, ball skills); (g) prehension and manipulation, and (h) motor planning. Each area has specific questions (total 182 on the observation guideline) that thoroughly address movement abilities. Observers are further permitted to address any other component within the area that they believe is pertinent. Age ranges for developmental motor milestones and an observation worksheet format are also provided in tables and figures to facilitate the assessment process.

Critique

This assessment provides a very thorough evaluation of the child's abilities in the major developmental domains and it can be linked easily to intervention. It is child-friendly because the environment is natural (i.e., a play setting), caregivers are involved in the testing, and only one professional must actively engage with the child.

TPBA does not provide comparison of the child to a normative population and therefore may not provide information required by states for child eligibility for special education services. For the adapted physical educator it does not provide an index of reflex involvement or an explanation of equilibrium responses. Additionally, time and scheduling constraints may make it difficult to participate in the arena style of testing. However, if the instrument is utilized as a component in determination of eligibility for services, the adapted physical educator may have time allocated for testing. Therefore time and scheduling may not be problematic and the TPBA would provide thorough information relative to many motor components.

Instrument Recommendations

Although one purpose of this chapter was to provide a theoretical model for assessment of infants, toddlers, and preschoolers, it is interesting to note that several of the instruments did not provide clear documentation of their theoretical framework. However, Bayley (1969) Ayres (1972, 1974, 1980) and Piaget (1954) were the predominant references cited as the theoretical basis for the design of several instruments. In the future, contemporary or revolutionary theorists (e.g., Thelen & Ulrich, 1991) will impact the focus and depth of intervention as the movement specialist continues to link assessment with intervention. There are several factors that must be considered by the interdisciplinary, transdisciplinary, or cross-disciplinary team when selecting and administering an assessment instrument (see Figure 5.22).

The model presented in Chapter 1 depicted the interaction of theory, assessment, and practice or intervention. Furthermore, the purpose of assessment and the ultimate goals and resultant programming for an individual should guide the examiner in the selection process. Initial considerations are the child's age, disability, severity of the condition, and family needs. Other considerations include: (a) the thoroughness of the instrument, (b) examiner qualifications, (c) time and feasibility for administration, (d) technical adequacy, and (e) the setting for administration (Van Deusen & Brunt, 1997).

The thoroughness of the instrument refers to the number of items the instrument evaluates in different motor categories. A thorough instrument would include, but not be limited to assessment of: (a) reflexes; (b) muscle tone; (c) balance, equilibrium, and postural control; (d) attainment of locomotor motor milestones; (e) evidence of associated reactions and unequal muscle tone during activity; (f) visual tracking; (g) eye-hand coordination in reach; (h) sensory systems analysis; (i) grasp; (j) release; (k) toy and object handling skills; and (1) interactive play behaviors. Based on the critical review of assessment instruments, recommendations for infants, toddlers, and preschoolers with disabilities are included within several categories: (a) determining eligibility, (b) educational programming, (c) use in various settings, and (d) examiner's professional expertise.

The Denver II (Frankenburg et al., 1992) and the Bayley Scales of Infant and Toddler Development (Third Edition) (Bayley III) (Bayley, 2006) are recommended for use with infants and toddlers in the process of determining eligibility for services. Although originally designed for screening, the Denver II is considered adequate for determining eligibility of infants and toddlers because it is standardized and provides a time-efficient evaluation of infant and toddler behavior. It can be used periodically to measure developmental gains. The Bayley III is a more thorough standardized assessment for infants and toddlers. It can be administered within a half hour with minimal equipment and provides normative data. When more in-depth assessment is desired, the Brigance Inventory of Early Development II (Brigance, 2004), and the Early Intervention Development Profile (Rogers & D'Eugenio, 1981) are also recommended.

Eligibility criteria for providing services to preschoolers is more strict and definitive than for infants and toddlers; therefore, the Battelle Developmental Inventory II (Newborg et al., 2004) is recommended for this age group. It is a comprehensive, standardized, norm-referenced assessment battery. The Early Intervention Developmental Profile (Rogers & D'Eugenio, 1981) is also recommended for use with preschoolers who have moderate to severe motor disabilities.

For educational programming, the Hawaii Early Learning Profile Charts and Activity Guide (Furuno et al., 2005) and the Early Intervention Development Profile (Rogers & D'Eugenio, 1981) are highly recommended for use with infants and toddlers. The preambulatory section of the Brigance Inventory (Brigance, 2004) and the Carolina Curriculum for Infants and Toddlers with Special Needs (Second Edition) (Johnson-Martin et al., 1991) are also recommended for children with severe disabilities. For children at the preschool level, the Brigance Inventory allows the professional to easily develop individual educational objectives. Although the Transdisciplinary Play-Based

Assessment (Linder, 1993) provides a thorough description of child abilities and links assessment with intervention, it is often not feasible for the movement specialist to participate in arena style assessment. However, with a modified format, the motor play phase of this assessment would provide thorough, useful information and is highly recommended for use with infants, toddlers, and preschoolers. Although not intended to be used in isolation it could provide excellent programming information.

The setting also impacts the selection of the assessment instrument. In the traditional educational setting, the Battelle Developmental Inventory (Newborg et al., 2004) and the Brigance Inventory (Brigance, 2004) are recommended. In a medical or hospital setting, the Denver II (Frankenburg et al., 1992) and the EIDP (Rogers & D'Eugenio, 1981) are suggested for use due to multiple time and space constraints of these settings. For the less experienced examiner, The HELP Checklist (Furuno et al., 1988) and HELP Strands (Parks, 2004) are recommended. They provide clear explanations, good sequencing, and hierarchy of items, and both have curricular applications.

SUMMARY

Definitions of assessment, the role of the movement specialist in a collaborative assessment process, a critical review of assessment instruments for infants, toddlers, and preschoolers, and recommendations for use by the movement specialist have been discussed. Each movement specialist must develop individual mechanisms for change to implement an action plan for assessment and intervention in their particular work environment. This chapter highlighted the necessity for the movement specialist to structure and explore paradigms within the motor assessment process.

REFERENCES

Auxter, D., Pyfer, J., & Huettig, C. (2005). *Principles and methods of adapted physical education and recreation* (10th ed.). New York: McGraw Hill.

Ayres, A. J. (1972). *Sensory integration and learning disorders.* Los Angeles: Western Psychological Services.

Ayres, A. J. (1974). Reading: A product of sensory integrative processes. In A.

Henderson, L. Lorens, E. Gilfoyle, C. Myers, & S. Prevel (Eds.), *The development of sensory integration theory and practice: A collection of the work of A. Jean Ayres* (pp. 167–175). Dubuque, IA: Kendall/Hunt. (Original work published 1968).

Ayres, A. J. (1980). *Sensory integration and the child.* Los Angeles: Western Psychological Services.

Bagnato, S. J., & Neisworth, J. T. (1990). *SPECS: System to Plan Early Childhood Services, Administration Manual.* Circle Pines, MN: American Guidance Service.

Bagnato, S. J., Neisworth, J. T., & Munson, S. M. (1989). *Linking developmental assessment and early intervention: Curriculum-based prescriptions.* Rockville, MD: Aspen.

Bayley, N. (1969). *The Calilfornia infant scale of motor development.* Berkeley: University of California.

Bayley, N. (2006). *Bayley scales of infant and toddler development* (3rd ed.). San Antonio, TX: Harcourt.

Bly, L. (1980). The components of movement during the first year of life. In *Development of movement in infancy.* Chapel Hill, NC: University of North Carolina, Division of Physical Therapy.

Bobath, B. (1948). The importance of the reduction of muscle tone and the control of mass reflex action in the treatment of spasticity. *Occupational Therapy, 27,* 371.

Bricker, D., Pretti-Frontczak, K., Johnson, J., & Straka, E. (2002). *AEPS Measurement for birth to three years, and three to six years, Administration Guide, Vol. 1.* Baltimore: Brookes.

Bricker, D., Capt, D., Pretti-Frontczak, K., & Johnson, J. (2002). *AEPS Measurement Tests, Vol. 2.* Baltimore: Brookes.

Bricker, D., & Waddell, M. (2002). *AEPS Curriculum for Birth to Three Years, Vol. 3.* Baltimore: Brookes.

Bricker, D., & Waddell, M. (2002). *AEPS Curriculum for Three to Six Years, Vol. 4.* Baltimore: Brookes.

Bricker, D., Squires, J., Mounts, L., Potter, L., Nickel, R., Twombly, E., & Farrell, J. (1999). *Ages and Stages Questionnaires: A Parent-Completed, Child-Monitoring System, Second Edition.* Baltimore: Brookes.

Brigance, A. H. (2004). *Brigance diagnostic inventory of early development II.* North Billerica, MA: Curriculum Associates.

Chandler, L. S., Andrews, M. S., & Swanson, M. S. (1980). *Movement assessment of infants: Manual.* Rolling Bay, WA: Infant Movement Research.

Cowden, J. E., & Eason, B. L. (1991). Pediatric adapted physical education for infants, toddlers and preschoolers: Meeting IDEA-H and IDEA-B challenges. *Adapted Physical Activity Quarterly, 8,* 263–279.

Cowden, J. E., & Sayers, L. K. (1997). Pediatric adapted motor development interactive assessment model. Unpublished manuscript. University of New Orleans, Department of Human Performance and Health Promotion with Children's Hospital, Department of Neurology and Neuroscience. New Orleans, LA.

Cowden , J. E., & Torrey, C. C. (1995). A ROADMAP for assessing infants, toddlers, and preschoolers: Role of the adapted motor developmentalist. *Adapted Physical Activity Quarterly, 12,* 1–11.

D'Eugenio, D. B., & Moersch, M. S. (Eds.) (1981). *Developmental programming for infants and young children: Preschool developmental profile.* Ann Arbor: University of Michigan Press.

Einarsson-Backes, L. M., & Stewart, K. B. (1992). Infant neuromotor assessments: A review and preview of selected instruments. *The American Journal of Occupational Therapy, 46*(3), 224–231.

Folio, M. R., & Fewell, R. B. (2000). *Peabody developmental motor scales and activity cards.* Austin, TX: Pro-ed.

Frankenburg, W. K., Dodds, J., Archer, P., Bresnick, B., Maschka, P., Edelman, N., & Shapiro, H. (1992). *Denver II* (2nd ed.). Denver, CO: Denver Developmental Materials.

Furuno, S., O'Reilly, K. A., Hosaka, C. M., Inatsuka, T. T., Alman, T. L., & Zeisloft, B. (2005). *HELP: Hawaii early learning profile charts and activity guide.* Palo Alto, CA: VORT.

Furuno, S., O'Reilly, K. A., Hosaka, C. M., Inatsuka, T. T., Zeisloft-Falbey, B., & Allman, T. L. (1988). *HELP Checklist: Ages birth to three years.* Palo Alto, CA: VORT.

Greenspan, S. I. (1992). *Infancy and early childhood: The practice of clinical assessment and intervention with emotional and developmental challenges.* Madison, CT: International University Press.

Henderson, S. E. (1994). Editorial. *Adapted Physical Activity Quarterly, 11*(2), 111–114.

Horvat, M. (2003). *Developmental/Adapted physical education: Making ability count* (4th ed.). San Francisco: Benjamin Cummings.

Horvat, M., & Kalakian, L. (1996). *Developmental/adapted physical education: Making ability count* (4th ed.) San Francisco: Benjamin Cummings.

Howard, V. F., Williams, B. F., Port, P. D., & Lepper, C. (1997). *Very young children with special needs: A formative approach for the 21st century.* Upper Saddle River, NJ: Merrill.

Johnson-Martin, N. M., Jens, K. G., Attermeier, S. M., & Hacker, B. J. (2004). *The Carolina curriculum for preschoolers with special needs.* Baltimore: Brookes.

Johnson-Martin, N. M., Jens, K. G., Attermeier, S. M., & Hacker, B. J. (2004). *The Carolina curriculum for infants and toddlers with special needs* (2nd ed). Baltimore: Brookes.

Linder, T. (1993). *Transdisciplinary play-based assessment* (Rev. ed.). Baltimore: Brookes.

Neisworth, J. T. (Ed.) (1990). Judgment-based assessment [Topical issue]. *Topics in Early Childhood Special Education, 16*(3).

Newborg, J., Stock, J., Wnek, L., Guidubaldi, J., & Svinicki, J. S. (2004). *Battelle developmental inventory* (2nd ed.) (BDI-2). Itasca, IL: Riverside Publishing.

Parks, S. (1999). *HELP when the parent has disabilities.* Palo Alto, CA: VORT.

Parks, S. (Ed.) (2004). *HELP strands: Curriculum-based developmental assessment birth to three years.* Palo Alto, CA: VORT.

Parks, S. (2006). *Inside HELP: Administration and reference manual.* Palo Alto, CA: VORT

Parks, S., Furuno, S., O'Reilly, K. A., Inatsuka, T. T., Hosaka, C. M., & Zeisloft-Falbey, B. (1995). *HELP at home.* Palo Alto, CA: VORT.

Piaget, J. (1954). *The construction of reality in the child.* New York: Basic Books.

Pikler, E. (1971). Learning of motor skills on the basis of self-induced movements. In J. Helmuth (Ed.), *Exceptional infant, Vol. 2. Studies in abnormalities*. New York: Brunner Mazel.

Rogers, S. J., Donovan, C. M., D'Eugenio, D., Brown, S. L., Lynch, E. W., Moersch, M. S., & Schafer, S. Ed (1981). *Developmental Programming for Infants and Young Children. Vol. 2. Early Intervention Developmental Profile*. Revised. Ann Arbor University of Michigan Press.

Rood, M. (1954). Neurophysiological reactions as a basis for physical therapy. *Physical Therapy Review, 34,* 444.

Rossetti, L. (1990). *Infant-toddler assessment: An interdisciplinary approach*. Boston: College-Hill Press.

Schaefer, D. S., & Moersch, M. S. (1981). *Developmental programming for infants and young children: Early intervention developmental profile*. Ann Arbor: University of Michigan Press.

Sherrill, C. (1993). *Adapted physical activity, recreation and sport: Crossdisciplinary and lifespan* (4th ed.). Madison, WI: Brown & Benchmark.

Sherrill, C. (1997, May). *Adaptation theory: Epistomological perspectives*. Paper presented at the meeting of the 11th International Symposium for Adapted Physical Activity, Quebec City, Canada.

Sherrill, C. (2004). *Adapted physical activity, recreation, and sport: Cross disciplinary and lifespan* (6th ed.). New York: McGraw-Hill.

Thelen, E., & Ulrich, B. D. (1991). Hidden skills: A dynamic systems analysis of treadmill stepping during the first year. *Monographs of the Society for Research in Child Development, 56, 1,* (Serial No. 223).

Van Deusen, J., & Brunt, D. (1997). *Assessment in occupational therapy and physical therapy*. Philadelphia, PA: W. B. Saunders.

VORT Corporation (1995). *HELP for Preschoolers Checklist*. Palo Alto, CA.

VORT Corporation (1999). *HELP for Preschoolers assessment and curriculum guide*. Palo Alto, CA.

VORT Corporation (2004). *HELP for Preschoolers assessment strands*. Palo Alto, CA.

Weschler, D. (2002). Weschler Preschool and Primary Scale of Intelligence (WPPSI). San Antonio, TX: The Psychological Corporation. Harcourt Assessment, Inc.

Widerstrom, A. H., Mowder, B. A., & Sandall, S. R. (1991). *At-risk and handicapped newborns and infants: Development, assessment, and intervention*. Englewood Cliffs, NJ: Prentice-Hall.

Wolery, M., & Dyk, L. (1984). Arena assessment: Description and preliminary social validity data. *Journal of the Association for the Severely Handicapped, 9*(3), 231–235.

Zittel, L. L. (1994). Gross motor assessment of preschool children with special needs: Instrument selection considerations. *Adapted Physical Activity Quarterly, 11* (3), 245–260.

Chapter 6

PRINCIPLES OF INTERVENTION:
PROGRESSIVE INTERACTIVE FACILITATION

Chapter Objectives: After studying this chapter, the reader will be able to:
1. Discuss the need for analyzing movement sequences for the development of individualized motor interventions for young children with motor delay;
2. Discuss the Progressive Interactive Facilitation theory;
3. Describe the 14 intervention principles of Progressive Interactive Facilitation and their implementation;
4. Delineate the progression of balance development;
5. Describe the establishment of gait patterns as delineated in the Progressive Model of Infant Stepping Movements;
6. Calculate the effects of an intervention program.

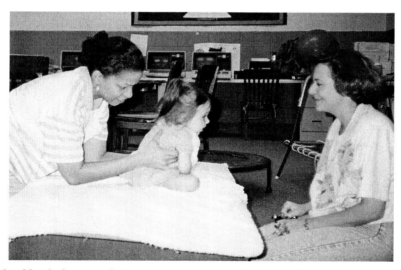

Figure 6.1. Vestibular stimulation assists in the development of muscle tone and balance that is required for independent sitting.

THEORETICAL PRINCIPLES OF INTERVENTION

The sensory and motor systems of the infant are intricately related and dependent upon each other. The baby learns through sensory stimulation gained mainly through the process of active and dynamic movement. The child develops the ability to lift his head and trunk against gravity, maintain a stable sitting and standing posture against gravity, and move without losing postural stability and balance.

During this process, motor control is initiated through the lower centers of the nervous system experiencing an inhibitory process, while higher levels of cortical control are modifying motor responses into new and more mature patterns of movement. Basically, the nervous system "learns by doing." The sensory input information (e.g., tactile, kinesthetic, visual, vestibular, and auditory) is received and transmitted by the nervous system, integrated at appropriate levels, and transmitted into motor actions, patterns, and movements. The elaborate system of interconnecting neurons, synaptic connections, afferent and efferent nerve pathways, and brain centers allow for the continued, sequential development of motor skills of the young child. Increasing sensorimotor maturity may be characterized by the dissociation of movement patterns involving the total body into selective and intricate parts of movements allowing for separate and independent actions of body parts. For example, the child can move one hand and arm without associated reaction occurring on the other side of the body or a child can stand on one foot without extraneous arm, body, or facial movements (see Figure 6.2).

It is necessary for movement sequences to be analyzed to determine exactly what may be causing motor delays (Sherrill, 1986). When a child is delayed in obtaining a sitting posture, what factors of muscle tone, strength, balance, and motor control are involved? The cause may influence the teaching strategies used with intervention. Intervention programs developed for young children should be based on theoretical principles which provide a directional structure.

Utilizing ideas from both medical and educational philosophies and principles that relate to normal and abnormal development, a program of exercises and activities for young children was designed. This Progressive Interactive Facilitation (PIF) theory proposes the following assumptions which relate to intervention in the motor domain: (a) neurodevelopmental facilitation and proprioceptive stimulation

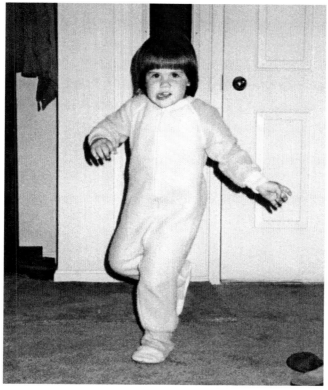

Figure 6.2. The presence of tongue protrusion and partial arm extensor and flexor pattern changes demonstrates the physiological stress this child is experiencing as she practices a challenging task.

through repetitive activities; (b) sequential interactive progression of exercises to facilitate the development of muscle tone, strength, and balance; (c) intersensory modality activation of motor output and feedback response; (d) progression of balance development; and (e) a progressive model of infant stepping movements.

Psychomotor developmental skill improves as primitive patterns are inhibited and more complex reactions are facilitated. The use of the word "skill" may seem awkward; however, Cratty (1964) defined the facilitation of skill as, "some learning has taken place or an integration of behavior has resulted" (p. 23). Combining this definition of skill with certain aspects of developmental fitness, the term "Specificity of Skill" has emerged as a major component for intervention. Exercises must be specific to the areas of the body (e.g., neck, trunk, arms, legs) and to specific muscle groups that need to be strengthened or relaxed

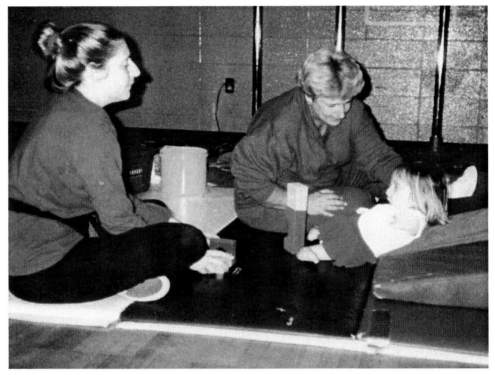

Figure 6.3. The movement specialist applies the specificity of skill approach to an exercise which increases the trunk strength of this infant with multiple congenital anomalies.

(see Figure 6.3).

More recently, Liemohn and Surburg (1997) presented considerations for the relationship of trunk muscle strength and essentials of flexibility. It is important to apply the concepts "muscle isolation for strength" and "muscle isolation for flexibility." Surburg (1997) further elaborated that "neuro-learning" and "neuro-transfer" are important to establishing smooth, efficient patterns of movement. Originally, Sherrington (1906) referred to the perception of sensation and the individual's own movement as the interactive component. Therefore, in the implementation of PIF, the interventionist must focus his/her thinking on the child's muscles which initiate the specific action desired. This may require the combination of hands-on facilitation of guided and coactive movements.

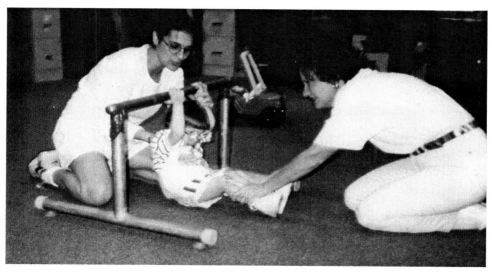

Figure 6.4. The interventionist assists an infant with Down syndrome and his mother with an exercise to increase muscle tone and strength.

INTERVENTION PRINCIPLES

Early intervention is the key to assisting infants and preschoolers with delays or disabilities. Families, as well as specialists in various developmental areas are critical in this intervention process (see Figure 6.4). As noted by theorists and interventionists (Gershkoff-Stowe & Thelen, 2004), children frequently perform more poorly before they do better. Therefore, during intervention, the movement specialist and families should expect regression before progression in developing movement behaviors. However, this is not truly regression, but the child's attempt to self-regulate his behavior and coordinate the components of the task and the environment.

During skill development/intervention sessions, the following key principles of PIF are recommended. They can be followed in home-based, center-based, and individualized motor sessions. The principles expound on the five theoretical assumptions that have been previously stated. A Progression of Balance Development, another component of PIF, is delineated later in the chapter.

1. Increase or decrease of muscle tone to facilitate effective movement

With some motor delays it is necessary for the interventionist to facilitate movements to increase muscle tone and strength. With other types of motor delays it is necessary to perform activities to inhibit muscle excitation and tension. The muscle tone of the newborn infant is predominantly flexor tone and development of extension gradually occurs in 2–3 months. The infant's inability to hold his or her head up in the prone position is an example of flexor tone dominance in the newborn.

2. Inhibition of primitive reflexes

Precautions should be taken to prevent the stimulation of primitive reflexes due to improper handling and positioning of children. Certain reflexes which are normal in the first 4–6 months should gradually disappear or be inhibited by the central nervous system. When a child's development has been delayed, it may be necessary to perform exercises which inhibit primitive patterns. Retention of primitive reflexes interfere with more mature forms of mobility.

3. Reciprocal innervation

Reciprocal innervation may be defined as the interaction of muscles contracting while the opposite muscles stretch or relax allowing for freedom of movement of bones and joints (see Figure 6.5). If an infant has retention of primitive reflexes, this component for facilitation of movement is compromised and the child lacks a smooth flow of efficient muscular actions.

4. Neurodevelopmental repetitive facilitation of movements

Repetitive sensorimotor stimulation may be necessary to facilitate actions or movements of immature nervous system pathways often found in children with disabilities (see Figure 6.6). Sensory inputs elicit motor output as a reflex, reaction or motor skill (Sherrill, 2004). Intersensory integration is also promoted by providing repetitive movements.

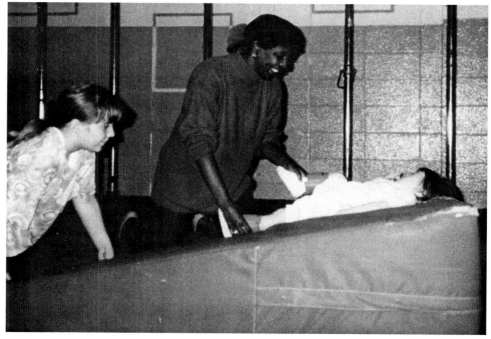

Figure 6.5. During the Pedal Pump exercise (see Chapter 7) one lower extremity relaxes as the other contracts during reciprocal innervation. Here, the addition of ankle weights and the effect of gravity facilitate acquisition of muscle tone and strength.

5. Stimulation of automatic equilibrium reactions

Specific exercises which increase muscle tone, strength, and balance allow for movements to stimulate the development of equilibrium reactions (see Figure 6.7). The vestibular, tactile, kinesthetic, and visual modalities should be stimulated through activities requiring rolling, tilting, and swinging.

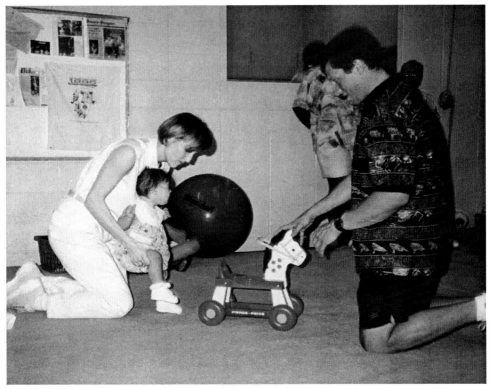

Figure 6.6. The principles of reciprocal innervation and neurodevelopmental repetitive facilitation are applied to this activity for facilitation of independent walking.

6. Tactile stimulation for warm-up, flexibility, range of motion, and relaxation

Warm-up is also necessary for young children to perform effective patterns of movement by raising the temperature and increasing circulation of the muscles and joints (see Figure 6.8). Flexibility, a health-related component of physical fitness, is specific to individual joints. Gentle range of motion and deep pressure massage promote elasticity of soft tissue which enables the child to perform some movements that might otherwise be impossible or extremely difficult to perform.

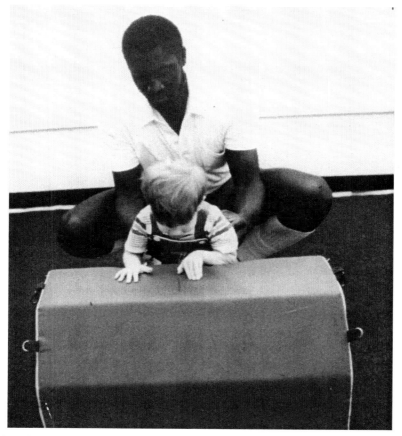

Figure 6.7. The movement specialist provides an exercise for stimulation of a child's equilibrium reactions through sensory stimulation.

7. Positioning for increasing muscle tone, strength, and balance of specific muscles

Strength is defined as the force exerted by muscles in a single contraction. The ability of muscles to sustain repeated contractions is termed **muscular endurance**. When muscle tone or muscular firmness is developed, strength is usually maintained or increased. Through sequences of exercises in various positions, muscle tone and strength are also developed leading to improved balance (see Figure 6.9). As movement efficiency improves, the infant spends less physiological or energy cost and overall quality of movement patterns improve.

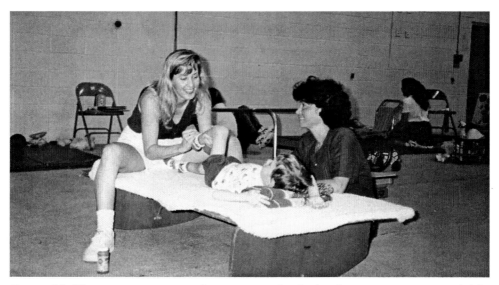

Figure 6.8. The interventionist implements an individualized warm-up prior to a child's pediatric strength intervention.

8. Coordination of stability and mobility

A blending of **stability** (holding strategies) and **mobility** (active movement) is necessary for upright locomotion. It is necessary to have a balanced distribution of tone or tension for static or mobile movements. Basically, walking is a developed skill of losing one's balance and regaining it while maintaining an upright position. Clumsy or unbalanced movements can be attributed to unequal muscle tone and lack of coordination during periods of stability and mobility.

9. Resistance training

With an increase in resistance to movements, muscle tone and strength increase. Hypotonia or weak muscle tone is a condition that may or may not involve central nervous system damage. Frequently, all central nervous system mechanisms are intact and hypotonia is a result of other syndromes or conditions. Sensory input or stimulation results in increased motor output or movement. Therefore, through the use of light ankle weights (e.g., quarter-pound or half-pound) resistance is increased and muscle tissue is developed. When muscle tissue replaces fatty tissue, muscle tone and strength can be increased.

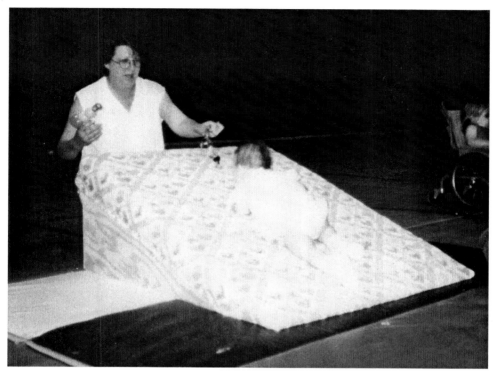

Figure 6.9. A mother demonstrates use of homemade equipment to implement the exercise "Crawling Up an Incline" (see Chapter 7) for increasing muscle tone, strength, and balance.

Specific combinations of exercises should be performed to strengthen the total body from head to toe (see Figure 6.10).

Weights or resistance training should be used very carefully with a child who has hypertonia or excessive muscle tone. The identification of flexed versus extensor tone dominance or abductor versus adductor tone dominance should be clearly established prior to using resistance training as a part of an early intervention program. A balance of weak versus strong muscle groups must be obtained to establish a smooth, efficient pattern of movement. For example, a child who presents fisted or flexed fingers should never be asked to squeeze a soft rubber ball to increase flexor tone strength because the flexor pattern is dominant and therefore is interfering with the quality of fine motor manipulation. The flexor muscle group should be relaxed/stretched by pressing the palm of the hand and extended fingers flat against a 4–6" playground ball.

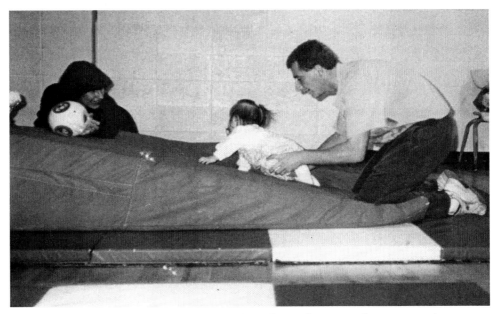

Figure 6.10. The child's interventionist and mother utilize an incline to provide a resistance exercise during hands-on facilitation of creeping.

10. Exercise sequences, repetitions, and sets

Exercises should be performed to develop flexion, extension, adduction, abduction, and rotational movements of various muscle groups. **Repetitions** are the number of times a muscle is required to contract during a specific exercise. **Sets** are the number of times an exercise should be repeated. Through muscle repetitions and increased sets, central nervous system excitation increases the transmission of nerve impulses necessary for the development of muscular strength and motor skill.

11. Frequency, duration, and rest

Frequency is how often an exercise is performed, **duration** is how long an exercise is performed and rest is required of muscle groups to prevent fatigue. **Exerted effort** is a positive term used to assist caregivers with understanding these concepts. The movement specialist should assist caregivers with determining the child's exercise sequences, repetitions, sets, frequency, duration, and rest when designing and monitoring individualized home-based pediatric strength interventions.

12. Overload, progression, and maintenance

It is necessary to have a progressive increase in resistance, exercise time, or repetitions for the development of muscle tone and increased strength. Careful monitoring of an infant's progress by the movement specialist and caregivers is necessary to make positive changes in the intervention program. Precautions should always be taken to ensure the safety of the child.

13. Dynamic action and adaptation

Theoretically, dynamic action implies a systematic relationship of internal biological changes with external environmental interactions (Thelen & Smith, 1994). The learning and exercise environment is an integral part of the exercise program. Movement provides the opportunity for learning experiences and can be considered the "language of intervention." Adaptation provides the process that allows for the exchange of internal and external information, therefore establishing the child's relationship with his/her surroundings. Without opportunities for movement, the child does not have a means to adapt to his or her environment.

14. Psychophysiological Response to Stress (PRS)

The challenge of attaining sequential movement skills by infants with delay or disability may cause adverse or negative elements of psychophysiological responses to stress. There is evidence to suggest that emotional reactions can interfere with neurological, cardiovascular, respiratory, and physiological processing (Bruess, 1994; Floyd, Mimms, & Yelding-Howard, 1995; National Center for Clinical Infant Programs, 1995). For example, a young child with delays or disabilities may compensate in one way or the other to accomplish a task. If hypotonia is present, the child may experience difficulty in moving to obtain a toy. As a result, negative patterns such as locking of the knees, ankles, or hips may be used to facilitate moving. An example for a child with hypertonicity may be that of regressing to primitive reflex control when challenged with the achievement of higher developmental skills. Butler and Cowden (1991) explored the benefits of tactile stimulation with children who exhibited hypertonicity. This research suggested relaxation techniques should also be considered as a therapeutic intervention. In addition, PRS may be measured by changes in the child's cardiovascular and respiratory systems and through judgment-based and observational assessment.

PROGRESSION OF BALANCE DEVELOPMENT

Another component of PIF is the delineation of balance development (see Figure 6.11)

Balance development begins by establishing a static proprioceptive or vestibular pattern in a stable position with accurate visual feedback for environmental interpretation. This visual sensory information allows the child to use exploratory patterns of movements which increase joint stability. Through initial motor assessment the child's abilities must be determined prior to intervention programming (Williams, 1983). Task indicators of overall efficiency of body movements, stability of base of support, body position, number of support limbs, and nature of support surfaces are assessed. For successful attainment of independent upright locomotion (i.e., walking), balance development must include adequate strength of postural muscles including extensor and flexor muscle groups, refinement of automatic reactions, and intersensory integration of the visual, kinesthetic, and vestibular modalities.

An extensive comparison of the individual measurement items of many assessment instruments for infants and young children (see Table 5.1, pp. 158–160) was completed to determine the most highly used motor "milestones" for determining progression to upright locomotion. The task analysis was developed due to inadequate identification throughout assessment instruments of prerequisite abilities or skills for the attainment of the developmental milestone of "walking." The assessment items appearing on the Progression of Balance Development provide a guide for the development of balance and walking.

PROGRESSION OF BALANCE DEVELOPMENT
FOR INFANTS AND TODDLERS

1. Head control–Lifts head to 45 degrees momentarily (0–3 mos)

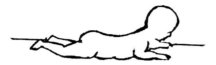

2. Head, neck, and shoulder muscles interacting (1–3 mos)

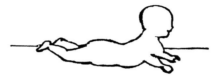

3. Lifts head, extends arms, and raises trunk (2–4 mos)

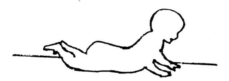

4. CNS integration of primitive reflexes (4–6 mos)

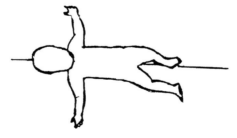

5. Rolls prone to side, to supine (4–6 mos)

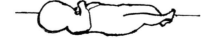

6. Sits momentarily leaning on hands (4–6 mos)

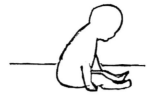

7. Sits independently without support (7–9 mos)

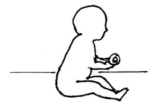

8. Equilibrium reactions matured (6–11 mos)

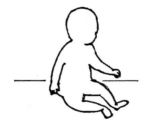

9. Pulls to standing (6–9 mos)

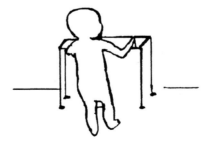

10. Crawls dragging body backward and forward (7–9 mos)

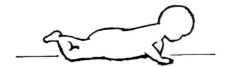

11. Creeps on hands and knees (9–11 mos)

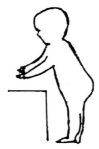

12. Stands unsupported for a few seconds (11–i3 mos)

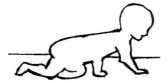

13. Walks with hands held (10–13 mos)

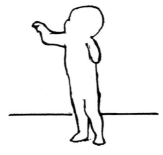

14. Walks without support (13–15 mos)

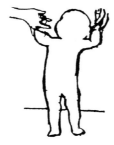

Figure 6.11. Progression of Balance Development for infants and toddlers.

PROGRESSIVE MODEL OF INFANT STEPPING MOVEMENTS

Traditional periods from infancy to toddlerhood are often determined according to the timelines in which the infant acquires walking skills (Bayley, 2006; Gesell, 1949; McGraw, 1932). It is such a significant motor milestone that the acquisition of upright locomotor patterns appears on most formal developmental assessment instruments used with young children. Although researchers differ on the specific time lines, an infant without disabilities usually acquires the skills to walk with support at approximately 12 months of age and to walk independently at approximately 13 months of age. Research reports a delayed acquisition of motor skills by infants with Down syndrome when compared to their nondisabled peers (Ulrich, Ulrich, & Collier, 1992). Infants with Down syndrome do not acquire walking skills until 13–48 months of age (Henderson, 1986; Ulrich &Ulrich, 1993; Ulrich et al., 1992).

Clark, Whitall, and Phillips (1988) studied human interlimb coordination during the first six months of independent walking. The focus of the research was on "understanding the nature of the interlimb organization evidenced in those first walking steps as well as possible changes in that organization as the infant practices walking for the next few months" (page 445). Most recently, Clark (2005) determined that a developmental perspective is critical to one's understanding of a person's movement and mobility: as one analyzes an individual's motor behavior, one must consider the importance of past movement experiences.

Infants with Down syndrome are faced with the additional complications of joint laxity and hypotonicity that are not experienced by infants without disabilities when attaining upright locomotor posture. Therefore, the progressive gaits of infants with Down syndrome are uniquely different from the progressive gaits of infants without disabilities. The final component of PIF involved the design of a new gait model for infants with hypotonia or Down syndrome (see Figure 6.12).

During a research study (Sayers, Cowden, Newton, Warren, & Eason, 1996) of infants with Down syndrome who participated in individualized pediatric strength interventions, it was recognized that the gaits of infants with Down syndrome could not be described according to existing models of infants who had attained independent upright locomotion (i.e., Auxter, Pyfer, & Huettig, 2005; Breniere & Do, 1991;

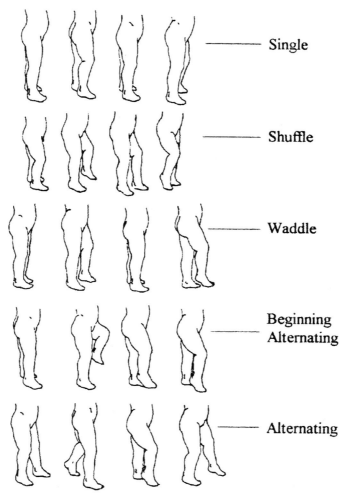

Single

Shuffle

Waddle

Beginning
Alternating

Alternating

Figure 6.12. Progressive Model of Infant Stepping Movements.

Shumway-Cook, Gallahue, & Ozmun, 1995; Sherrill, 1993; Shumway, Cook & Woollacott, 1985; Thelen & Cooke, 1987; Thelen, Ulrich, & Jensen, 1989; and Ulrich et al., 1992) (see Figure 6.13). If the infant did not have the movement potential for step initiation, then the traditional phase descriptions of heel strike, midstance, pushoff, and swing-through were not applicable. The Progressive Model of Infant Stepping Movements (see Table 6.1) was designed which allows for quantifying the measurements of an infant's step initiation, foot placement, stance, and swing phase (see Figure 6.14).

Table 6.1 Progressive Model of Infant Stepping Movements Data Recording Form.

Place a check beside the best description of the infant's stepping movements.

Subject No._____ Pretest:_____ Posttest:_____

Preanalysis Coding

Step Initiation Phase
1. knee lock of stepping foot
2. lifting of stepping foot
3. weight placement remains on support leg and foot
4. forward transfer of weight to stepping foot
5. hands grip parallel bars for balance
6. head up, eyes focused on destination or head down, eyes focused on feet
7. no trunk rotation or slight trunk rotation

Foot Placement to Stance Phase
1. a. *shuffle:* during weight shift to placement foot, placement foot is shuffled forward as it maintains contact with the surface
   b. *waddling:* weight shifts to placement foot as trunk leans in direction of weight shift with little knee and hip flexion
   c. *single:* knee lift and hip flexion lead to forward transfer of weight to stepping foot as homolateral steps are taken
   d. *alternating:* knee lift and hip flexion lead to forward transfer of weight to stepping foot as bilateral steps are taken

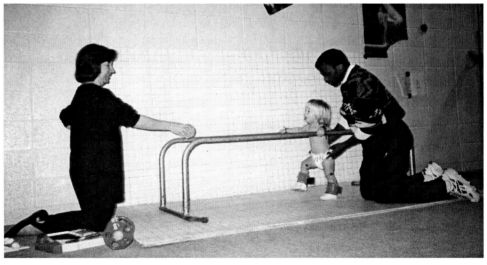

Figure 6.13. The mother and the movement specialist facilitate walking through pediatric parallel bars to allow this infant to support her body weight during guided steps toward a favorite toy.

2. a. arms slide along parallel bars in opposition
   b. arms move along parallel bars in opposition as hands are lifted from parallel bars and lowered back down to grip parallel bars
   c. arms are in highguard position not utilizing parallel bars for balance
   d. arms swing reciprocally with walk
3. a. head up, eyes on destination
   b. head down, eyes on feet
4. a. knees and feet are turned in
   b. knees and feet are turned out
   c. knees and feet are pointing forward
5. a. feet are in plantar flexion
   b. feet are in dorsiflexion
   c. feet are flat
6. a. no trunk rotation
   b. slight trunk rotation

Swing Phase
1. a. *shuffling:* swing leg is shuffled forward as swing foot maintains contact with ground
   b. *waddling:* swing leg is brought forward with little knee and hip flexion as trunk leans in direction of the swing leg side of the body
   c. *single:* knee lift and hip flexion of swing leg leads to lifting of swing foot, forward swing of limb, and contact of swing foot parallel to stationary foot; movements are homolateral
   d. *alternating:* knee lift and hip flexion of swing leg leads to lifting of swing foot, forward swing of limb and forward contact of swing foot to surface; movements are bilateral
2. a. arms slide along parallel bars in opposition
   b. arms move along parallel bars in opposition as hands are lifted from parallel bars and lowered back down to grip parallel bars.
   c. arms are in highguard position not utilizing parallel bars for balance
   d. arms swing reciprocally with walk
3. a. head up, eyes on destination
   b. head down, eyes on feet
4. a. knees and feet are turned in
   b. knees and feet are turned out
   c. knees and feet are pointing forward
5. a. feet are in plantar flexion
   b. feet are in dorsiflexion
   c. feet are flat
6. a. no trunk rotation
   b. slight trunk rotation

Identification of Step Types during walking
1. *shuffling:* both feet are alternately shuffled forward as they maintain contact with the surface
2. *waddling:* trunk leans to the side of the body from which alternating forward steps are taken in a waddling manner
3. *single:* steps occur in a single manner from only one side of the body (forward homolateral movement in a slide manner)

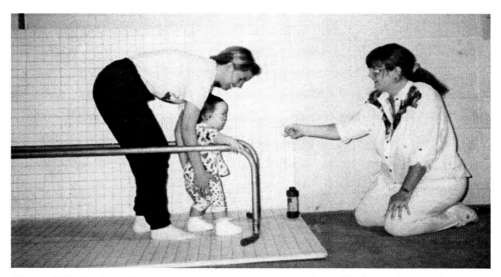

Figure 6.14. As the infant acquires muscle tone, strength, and balance, her guided walking patterns through the parallel bars (and later without support) can be analyzed according to the Progressive Model of Infant Stepping Movements.

4. *beginning alternating:* steps occur in an alternating manner from one foot to the other with slight forward movement (hands grip parallel bars)
5. *alternating:* steps occur in an alternating manner from one foot to the other with good forward movement (arms and hands initiate limited crosslateral arm movement with hands lifted from parallel bars)

This permits the movement specialist to describe the infant's gait as one of the following progressive step types from beginning upright stepping to a traditional walking pattern: (a) shuffle-both feet are alternately shuffled forward as they maintain contact with the surface during step initiation, foot placement to stance and swing phase of movement; (b) waddle-trunk leans to the side of the body from which alternating forward steps are taken with little knee and hip flexion during step initiation, foot placement to stance and swing phase of movement; (c) single-steps occur in a single manner from only one side of the body in a sliding manner; (d) beginning alternating-steps occur in an alternating manner from one foot to the other with slight forward movement; (e) alternating-steps occur in an alternating manner from one foot to the other with good forward movement.

IMPLEMENTATION AND EVALUATION OF PIF

The theoretical premises of PIF are best applied to home-based individualized pediatric strength interventions which involve the child, caregivers, and movement specialist in the design and implementation of the program. This approach focuses on caregiver involvement in assessment and intervention, thus acknowledging the caregiver as a reliable source of information (Beckman, 1984; Bricker & Squires, 1989; Gradel, Thompson, & Sheehan, 1981). Because the intervention is implemented in the natural context of the child's home environment, this design facilitates interaction between caregivers and child, utilizes the surroundings most comfortable for the child, allows the intervention to be implemented at times when the child is most alert, and increases caregiver knowledge and skills in the facilitation of motor development. A movement specialist working primarily in a center-based program can apply this approach to individual and group interventions implemented at the center as well as provide parent training for home-based implementation of the intervention.

A developmental assessment should be given prior to designing the intervention program. The assessment should utilize standardized and curriculum-based instruments along with judgment-based assessment and responses from an interview with the child's caregivers. The individually designed program should be based on the theoretical premises of PIF. A balance of the child's current abilities and progressive challenges should encourage each child's advancement to subsequent levels of motor development. The movement specialist should provide the caregivers with a written Pediatric Strength Intervention Performance Chart (see Table 6.2). Feedback from the caregivers and movement specialist's observations, hands-on evaluation, and judgment-based assessment should determine the frequency, intensity, mode, and duration of each exercise.

Table 6.2. Pediatric Strength Intervention Performance Chart.

Under the handwritten exercise prescription, record the frequency, sets, and repetitions as they are performed.

Child's Name:_____   Teacher:_____

Starting Date:_____   Ending Date:_____

Exercise_____	Freq/ Week	Sets	Reps
_____	_____	_____	_____
	_____	_____	_____
	_____	_____	_____
	_____	_____	_____
_____	_____	_____	_____
	_____	_____	_____
	_____	_____	_____
	_____	_____	_____
_____	_____	_____	_____
	_____	_____	_____
	_____	_____	_____
	_____	_____	_____

It is very important for the movement specialist to discuss with the family the appropriate guidelines for administering the home-based intervention and to continuously monitor the implementation of these guidelines. At a minimum, the guidelines should include the following: (a) an explanation of the exercise prescription including a demonstration by the movement specialist, the caregiver practicing of the exercises with the child, and an explanation of the frequency, set, and repetitions; (b) the importance of the child maintaining proper body alignment during the exercises; (c) properly adapting the necessary home or commercial equipment; (d) allowing the child to put forth exerted effort during the movements; (e) providing an atmosphere of fun and play during the implementation of the exercises; and (f) following the child's lead without continuously targeting a particular muscle group. In essence, the design and implementation of the program is very similar to the currently popular "personal trainer" employed to evaluate someone's physical fitness status and individualize a fitness routine to help the person achieve desirable fitness goals.

Many times interventionists must provide documentation as to the effectiveness of their programs. Two methods for quantifying a child's development during intervention have been utilized: intervention-developmental quotient and posttest developmental age compared to predicted developmental age (Fewell & Glick, 1996; Fewell & Oelwein, 1991; Oelwein, Fewell, & Pruess, 1985; Sayers et al., 1996; Snyder-McLean, 1987). Snyder-McLean (1987) proposed the intervention developmental quotient be calculated to determine the child's rate of progress during the intervention. A child's pretest developmental quotient can be calculated using a standardized evaluation during the initial assessment process. The pretest developmental quotient is calculated by dividing the child's developmental age (as determined by the standardized evaluation) by his chronological age. This pretest developmental quotient reflects the child's entire lifetime of learning from birth through the time of pretest. At the end of the intervention period for which progress or development must be shown the same standardized evaluation is given as a posttest. To calculate the child's intervention developmental quotient, subtract the child's pretest developmental age from the posttest developmental age and divide the difference by the length of intervention. The intervention developmental quotient can then be contrasted with the pretest developmental quotient.

Snyder-McLean (1987) suggested the following advantages to the intervention developmental quotient formula: (a) by acknowledging each child's pretest developmental quotient it allows for observable changes that may be attributable to maturation; (b) it "factors out the minimizing effects of increasing CA [chronological age] on the size of DQ [developmental quotient] gains associated with intervention" (p. 262); and (c) "this approach is simple and allows evaluation data to be presented to broad audiences in a meaningful way" (p. 262).

The intervention developmental quotient formula was used to determine the effects of a strength intervention program designed for infants with Down syndrome (Cowden, Sayers & Torrey, 1998; Sayers, et al., 1996). Pre and posttesting involved normative, curriculum-based, and judgment-based measures and video analysis of gait patterns. Eight-week interventions were completed in home-based programming to facilitate muscle tone, strength, and balance development. Intervention included exercise programs using a combination of neurodevelopmental patterning, intersensory modality stimulation, a task analysis approach to equilibrium, gait analysis and a sequential, interactive progression of exercises, in accord with the PIF intervention principles. The caregivers were trained in exercise implementation, positioning and handling, relaxation and stimulation, and the proper use of homemade and commercial equipment. The results of the data offered support for the application of the PIF principles for muscle tone, strength, and balance development of infants with delays or disabilities.

Fewell, and Glick (1996) employed the second suggested approach to determine the intervention effects of an early intervention program and to determine if there were differences in the effects of the intervention outcomes for children who were less impaired than those who were more impaired. They compared posttest developmental ages to predicted developmental ages. "The predicted developmental ages (in months) at posttest were computed by multiplying the pretest DQ [developmental quotient] (proportion) by the amount of time in intervention (in months) and then adding the result to the child's pretest developmental age" (p. 237). They summarized their calculations as follows:

> **Step 1:** Pretest Developmental Age in Months/Pretest CA (chronological age) in Months = Pretest DQ developmental quotient)
> **Step 2:** Pretest DQ x Months in Intervention = Predicted Months Gain
> **Step 3:** Predicted Months Gain + Pretest Developmental Age (months) = Predicted Developmental Age (in months) at Posttest

Statistical analysis was used to determine significant differences between predicted developmental ages and actual developmental ages of the subjects.

In their discussion of results, Fewell and Glick (1996) acknowledged the limitation of their formula for predicted gain ". . . being based upon the assumption that without intervention, children will develop linearly and at a constant rate" (p. 241). However, they point out the formula does account for individual trajectories. In light of their study and the difficulties in finding models which appropriately analyze gain, these researchers suggested, "Perhaps it is time for practitioners, program evaluators, and policymakers to seriously revisit the criteria and measurement for program effectiveness" (p. 239).

SUMMARY

This chapter provided an intervention theory from which professionals and caregivers can individualize motor development programs. Two models have been designed which should assist in delineating interventions into specific components and provide a better understanding of individual movement patterns. In addition, research data were summarized detailing the specific and individual changes of infants with Down syndrome, thus providing support for the theoretical intervention components of PIF.

REFERENCES

Auxter, D., Pyfer, J., & Huettig, C. (2005). *Adapted physical education and recreation* (10th ed.). New York: McGraw Hill.

Bayley, N. (2006). *Bayley scales of infant and toddler development* (3rd ed.). San Antonio, TX: Harcourt.

Beckman, P. (1984). Perceptions of young children with handicaps: A comparison of mothers and program staff. *Mental Retardation, 22,* 176–181.

Breniere, Y., & Do, M. C. (1991). Control of gait initiation. *Journal of Motor Behavior, 23* (4), 235–240.

Bricker, D. D., & Squires, J. (1989). The effectiveness of parental screening of at-risk infants: The infant monitoring questionnaires. *Topics in Early Childhood Special Education, 9* (3), 67–85.

Bruess, C. E. (1994). *Healthy decisions.* Madison, WI: Brown & Benchmark.

Butler, G., & Cowden, J. E. (1991). Tactile stimulation as therapeutic intervention for children with hypertonicity. *LAHPERD Journal, 53* (2), 27.

Clark, J. E. (2005). From the beginning: A developmental perspective on movement and mobility. *Quest, 57*(1), 37–45.

Clark, J. E., Whitall, J., & Phillips, S. J. (1988). Human interlimb coordination: The first 6 months of independent walking. *Developmental Psychobiology, 21*(5), 445–456.

Cowden, J. E., Sayers, L. K., & Torrey, C. C. (1998). *Pediatric adapted motor development and exercise: An innovative multisystem approach for families and professional.* Springfield: IL: Charles C Thomas.

Cratty, B. (1964). *Movement behavior and motor learning.* Philadelphia: Lea and Febiger.

Fewell, R. R., & Glick, M. P. (1996). Program evaluation findings of an intensive early intervention program. *American Journal on Mental Retardation, 101* (3), 233–243.

Fewell, R. R., & Oelwein, P. L. (1991). Effective early intervention: Results from the model preschool program for children with Down syndrome and other developmental delays. *Topics in Early Childhood Special Education, 11*(1), 56–68.

Floyd, P. A., Mimms, S. E., & Yelding-Howard, C. (1995). *Personal health: A multicultural approach.* Englewood, CO: Morton.

Gallahue, D. L., & Ozmun, J. C. (1995). *Understanding motor development: Infants, children, adolescents, adults* (3rd ed.). Dubuque, IA: Brown & Benchmark.

Gershkoff-Stowe, L., & Thelen, E. (2004). U-shaped changes in behavior: A dynamic systems perspective. *Journal of Cognition and Development, 5*(1), 11–36.

Gesell, A. (1949). *Gesell Developmental Schedules.* New York: Psychological Corp.

Gradel, K., Thompson, M. S., & Sheehan, R. (1981). Parental and professional agreement in early childhood assessment. *Topics in Early Childhood Special Education, 1,* 31–39.

Henderson, S. E. (1986). Some aspects of the development of motor control in Down's syndrome. In H. T. A. Whiting & M. G. Wade (Eds.), *Themes in motor development* (pp. 69–92), Boston: Martinus Nijhoff.

McGraw, M. B. (1932), From reflex to muscular control in the assumption of erect posture and ambulation in the human infant. *Child Development, 3,* 291–297.

National Center for Clinical Infant Programs (1995). *Diagnostic Classification of Mental Health and Developmental Disorders of Infancy and Early Childhood.* Arlington, VA: Zero To Three/National Center for Clinical Infant Programs, 2000 14th Street North, Suite 380.

Oelwein, P. L., Fewell, R. R., & Pruess, J. (1985). Efficiency of intervention at outreach sites of the program for children with Down syndrome and other developmental delays. *Topics in Early Childhood Special Education, 5,* 78–87.

Sayers, L. K., Cowden, J. E., Newton, M., Warren, B., & Eason, B. (1996). Qualitative analysis of a pediatric strength intervention on the developmental stepping movements of infants with Down syndrome. *Adapted Physical Activity Quarterly, 13* (3), 247–268.

Sherrill, C. (1986). *Adapted physical education and recreation: A multidisciplinary approach* (3rd ed.). Dubuque, IA: Wm. C. Brown.

Sherrill, C. (1993) *Adapted physical activity, recreation, and sport: Crossdisciplinary and lifespan* (4th ed.). Dubuque, IA: Brown & Benchmark.

Sherrill, C. (2004). *Adapted physical activity, recreation and sport: Crossdisciplinary and lifespan* (6th ed.). New York: McGraw Hill.

Sherrington, C. S. (1906). *The integrative action of the nervous system.* New Haven: Yale University.

Shumway-Cook, A., & Woollacott, M. H. (1985). Dynamics of postural control in the child with Down syndrome. *Physical Therapy, 65,* (9) 1315–1322.

Snyder-McLean, L. (1987). Reporting norm-referenced program evaluation data: Some considerations. *Journal of the Division of Early Childhood, 11,* 254–264.

Surburg, P., & Liemohn-Surburg, W. (1997). Considerations for the relationship of trunk muscle strength and essentials of flexibility. Presentation at the Research

Consortium Symposium of the American Alliance for Health, Physical Education, Recreation and Dance, St. Louis, MO.

Thelen, E., & Cooke, D. W. (1987). Relationship between newborn stepping and later walking: A new interpretation. *Developmental Medicine and Child Neurology, 29,* 380–393.

Thelen, E., & Smith, L. B. (1994). *A dynamic systems approach to the development of cognition and action.* Cambridge, MA: The MIT Press.

Thelen, E., Ulrich, B. D., & Jensen, J. L. (1989). The developmental origins of locomotion. In M.H. Woollacott & A. Shumway-Cook (Eds.), *Development of posture and gait across the lifespan* (pp. 25–47). Columbia: University of South Carolina.

Ulrich, B. D., & Ulrich, D. A. (1993). Dynamic systems approach to understanding motor delay in infants with Down syndrome. In G. J. P. Savelsbergh (Ed.), *The development of coordination in infancy.* Elsevier Science Publishers B.V.

Ulrich, B. D., Ulrich, D. A., & Collier, D. H. (1992). Alternating stepping patterns: Hidden abilities of 11-month-old infants with Down syndrome. *Developmental Medicine and Child Neurology, 34,* 233–239.

Williams, H. (1983). *Perceptual and motor skills.* Englewood Cliffs, NJ: Prentice-Hall.

Chapter 7

ACTIVITIES FOR CHILDREN
WITH HYPOTONICITY

Chapter Objectives: After studying this chapter, the reader will be able to:
1. Discuss the organization of space, scheduling, and environmental factors in providing intervention services to young children with atypical muscle tone, lack of reflex integration, sensory motor delays, and manipulative problems (see Chapters 7, 8, 9, 10);
2. Determine if a child is exhibiting too much muscle tone (hypertonicity), too little muscle tone (hypotonicity), or typical muscle tone;
3. Apply intervention principles to assessment information and design an individualized exercise and activity program for a young child with hypotonicity or lack of muscular strength.

INTRODUCTION TO
DEVELOPMENTAL ACTIVITY PROGRAMS

This second section of the text is designed to provide practical, hands-on activities for the professional and family. Each chapter addresses a specific deficit: hypotonicity, hypertonicity, sensory motor control, and fine motor/hand control. After determining the deficit areas and corresponding muscle groups that the child is having most difficulty with, engaging in these activities will facilitate more mature and functional forms of movement for the child. The activities are based on the theoretical principles of Progressive Interactive Facilitation, and are designed to develop muscle tone, strength, and motor control, and to facilitate development towards an improved level of mobility.

During assessment, the specialist must first determine if the child is exhibiting too little muscle tone (hypotonicity) or too much muscular tension (hypertonicity). Some infants with multisensory delays will demonstrate fluctuating tone. Often it is thought that if a young child has hypotonicity, he or she probably will not exhibit delayed primitive reflexes. Even though motor tone may be low, as in the case of infants with Down syndrome, an infant trying to accomplish new skills will often demonstrate delay in primitive reflex integration, especially with the tonic neck group of reflexes.

The teacher should provide guided and patterned assistance as needed to move the child through the exercises. By allowing the child to support weight through movements, the teacher can "feel" the muscle groups contract and follow the child's lead without continuously targeting a particular muscle group. Toys, bubbles, and music should be incorporated as part of the exercise program to provide an environment of fun, play, and reinforcement to the infant so he/she will want to participate in the activities.

Organization of one's teaching space is necessary to provide optimal programming for young children. In schools or infant/toddler/preschool centers, motor specialists are typically itinerant and move to several centers. Within a particular specialist's schedule, time frames are developed to visit all centers, and afterward the principal and teacher are consulted regarding the individual child's schedule. There are often interfering priorities and in reality, motor intervention may become secondary to cognitive or language intervention. It may be difficult to find a perfect fit between the specialist's and child's schedules, as well as finding an appropriate space at the center for the motor activities to occur during that time frame. An ideal space for motor activities is often unavailable, and teaching may occur in cramped spaces, without optimal equipment, and where distractions frequently occur.

Incorporating the exercises in the natural environment of the home or classroom setting and improvising as necessary provide the essential structure and progression of the movement program. At infant/toddler/preschool centers, teaching in the least restrictive environment is mandated by Individuals with Disabilities Education Improvement Act (IDEA) (2004) and teaching children with disabilities in an integrated setting with children who are typical is recommended. However, with children who are functioning at low motoric levels (functioning age below 8 months), one-to-one teaching with concentration on development of typical muscle tone, reflex integration, and sensory motor activities is needed. Once children progress to a motor functioning age of 9+ months, they can be paired or grouped to engage in more interactive play activities. Engagement in play with typical and other motor delayed peers in a typical setting should be encouraged.

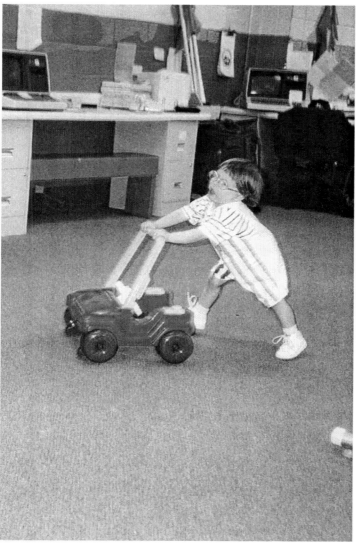

Figure 7.1. The activities in this chapter increase muscle tone and strength leading towards attainment of independent walking.

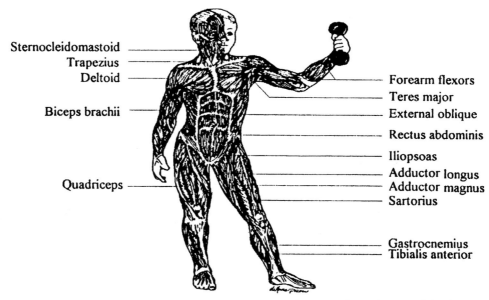

Figure 7.2. The primary muscle groups are identified for the frontal view of the human body. Exercises for these muscle groups in Chapters 7, 8, 9, and 10.

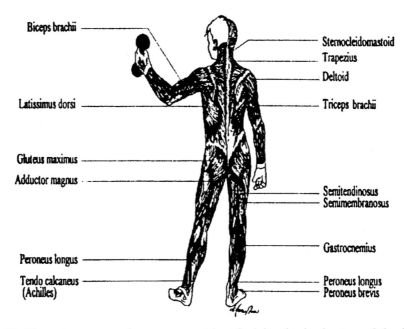

Figure 7.3. The primary muscle groups are identified for the back view of the human body. Exercises for these muscle groups are in Chapters 7, 8, 9, and 10.

EXERCISES AND ACTIVITIES FOR
INCREASING MUSCLE TONE AND STRENGTH

The exercises and activities are designed specifically for infants, toddlers, and preschoolers with delayed motor development who exhibit hypotonicity and lack of muscular strength. Activities and exercises are presented in sequence for the development of specific muscle groups according to head, neck, trunk, and extremities (see Figures 7.2 and 7.3), and lead to attainment of upright posture or walking. One must keep in mind the child's potential for achievement within the realm of the disability. Primary muscle groups which are involved in specific actions are also listed.

Hypotonia is exhibited if, when placed in the supine position, the infant lacks spontaneous movement, the legs are fully abducted and rotated outward with side of thigh lying flat against the surface (e.g., mat, table, floor), and the arms lie to the side either extended or flexed. When placed in a sitting position the head may fall forward with the shoulders limp and drooping.

Disabilities that often have behaviors relating to an infant with hypotonicity may include (a) chromosome disorders (e.g., Down syndrome, Prader-Willi syndrome); (b) prenatal distress or postnatal disorders; (c) metabolic disorders; (d) spinal cord disorders (e.g., injuries, hypoxic ischemia myelopathy); (e) spinal muscular atrophies (e.g., arthrogryposis, infantile and chronic infantile muscular disorders); (f) muscular dystrophies. The list is not a complete listing of congenital or infantile problems that may involve muscular weakness.

Supine Position

On back, arms at sides, palms of hands down, legs extended.

Motion Control: Head and neck flexion and extension
Muscle Groups: Sternocleidomastoid, upper trapezius, levator scapulae, splenius capitus, splenius cervicis.

Exercise 1: Look at Toes

Lift head and tuck chin to chest. Pull toes toward head (dorsiflex).

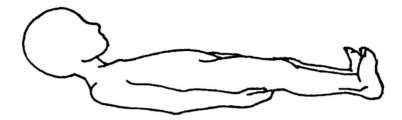

Exercise 2: Head Rotations

Turn the head slowly to right side and touch chin to shoulder, then to left side. If hands and arms move, press slightly down on palms of hands to maintain position.

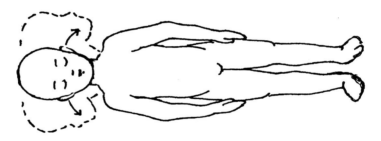

Motion Control: Neck, shoulders, trunk, and hip flexion.

Muscle Groups: Sternocleidomastoid, trapezius, rectus abdominis, internal and external obliques, rectus femoris.

Position: On back, knees bent, place child's arms across the child's chest. Do not pull child to sitting by pulling on extended arms. This could cause injury to the elbow and shoulder.

Exercise 3: Pediatric Sit-ups

Position the child on an incline wedge as needed for support to assist the child in raising the head and upper trunk toward the knees. Feet should remain flat on floor surface.

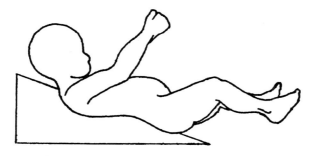

Motion Control:	Head, neck, trunk, hips, and legs.
Muscle Groups:	Additional muscle action: Quadriceps, hamstrings, adductors, gluteus muscles.
Position:	On back, knees bent.

Exercise 4: Pedal Pump

Kick legs in place using reciprocal pedal motion. May need to provide coactive assistance to help the child flex and extend the legs.

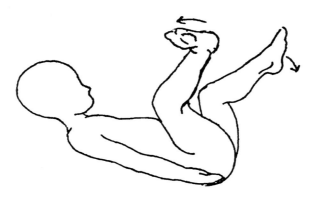

Exercise 5: Knee Pat

Raise arm/hand to touch lifted bent-knee on same side of body. Repeat on other side. Repeat by reaching across to opposite knee (see Figure 7.4).

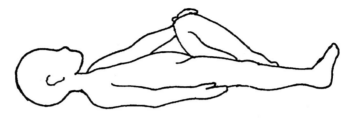

Motion Control: Shoulder, arm, wrist, and hand.
Muscle Groups: Pectoralis major and minor, rhomboid, deltoid, biceps, triceps, brachioradialis, and pronator teres and quadratus.

Exercise 6: Toy Pass

Lift arms and reach for the sky; pass favorite toy from one hand to other.

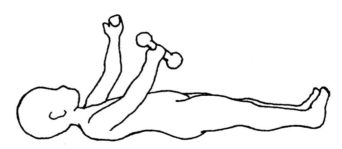

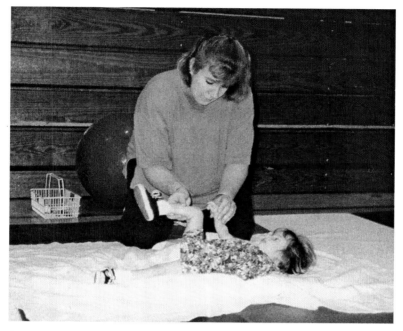

Figure 7.4. Exercise 5: This young girl is being assisted in completing a knee pat.

Exercise 7: Arm Flex

Flex arms to chest with hands to midline; stimulate child to turn head from side to side.

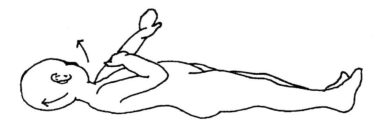

Motion Control:	Shoulders, arms, leg (adductor and abductor muscles).
Muscle Groups:	Deltoids, biceps, triceps, pectoralis major, latissimus dorsi, and adductor/abductor muscles of legs.

Exercise 8: Back Stroke

Move arms above head, flat on mat. Move legs apart at same time side to side.

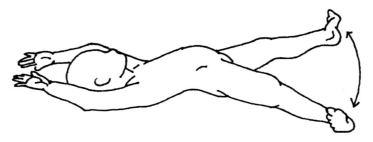

Motion Control: Trunk, hip flexion, and side-to-side rotation.

Exercise 9: Easter Egg Roll

Side-to-side roll like an egg.

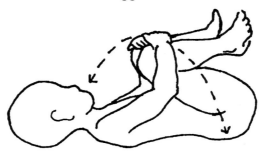

Exercise 10: Tuck Tight

Flex knees to chest in tuck position. Encourage the child to wrap the arms around the knees holding a tucked position.

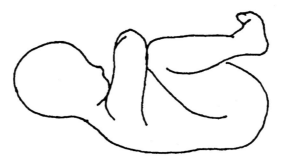

Exercise 11: Supine Rocker

Tuck chin to chest. Rock slowly back and forth.

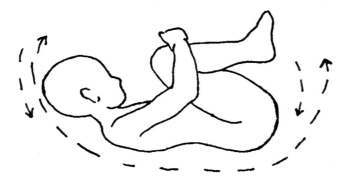

Motion Control: Arm and shoulder flexion and extension.

Exercise 12: Pull-up

Using low 12" bar, bent-knee position, pull up with arms. Placing the palms up on the bar works the biceps. Pulling up with arms (palms down) work with triceps.

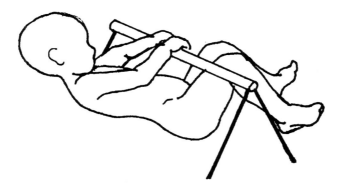

Motion Control: Hip and knee flexion.

Exercise 13: Knee Touch to Bar

Lift one knee at a time and bend to touch bar.

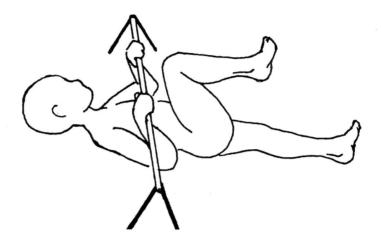

Motion Control: Head, trunk, and arm strength.

Exercise 14: Rope Pull

Pull child from floor keeping arms partially flexed at the elbow and hold away from mat momentarily; return slowly to supine position.

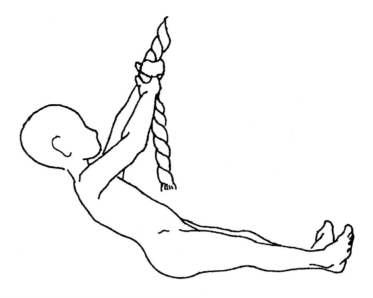

Motion Control: Head, trunk, and hip rotation.

Exercise 15: Extended Side Roll

Log-roll to side from supine, and back to other side.

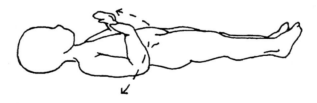

Prone Position

On stomach, legs extended, arms forward in prop position.

Motion Control: Head, neck, upper trunk, and arms.
Muscle Groups: Sternocleidomastoid, trapezius, pectoralis major and minor, biceps, triceps, deltoids, muscle groups of forearm.

Exercise 16: Prone Prop

Support under chest with small (i.e., 4"–5" wedge or bolster.
Lift head and neck and prop-up with hands and arms.
Visually stimulate with favorite toy (see Figure 7.5).

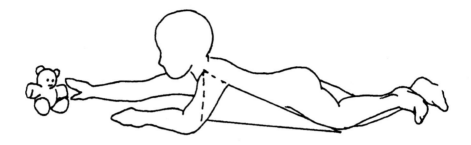

Exercise 17: Prone Reach

Move object/toy forward and encourage the child to extend
the arms slightly and reach for toy.

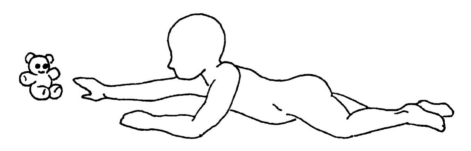

Motion Control:	Head, neck, trunk, arms, legs.
Muscle Groups:	Trapezius, latissimus dorsi, internal and external obliques, abdominals, deltoid, biceps, triceps, pectoralis major.

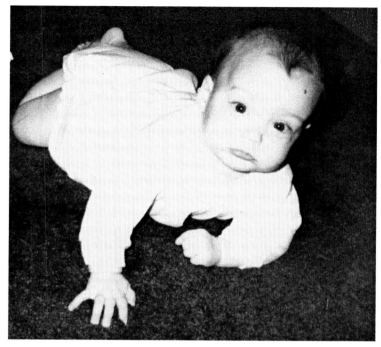

Figure 7.5. Exercise 16: The infant is pushing to the position of prone prop.

Exercise 18: Inchworm Reach

Child fully extends the arms and reaches forward. Encourage him/her to pull body forward as strength increases.

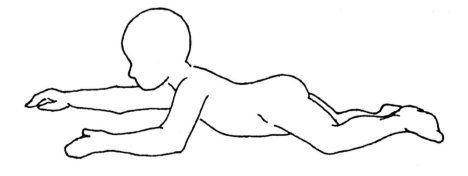

Motion Control: Head, neck, shoulders, trunk, arms, leg flexion and extension.

Exercise 19: Puppy Prop

Provide guided assistance by flexing knees and elbows of child. Support under trunk to allow for holding the 4-pt. position momentarily.

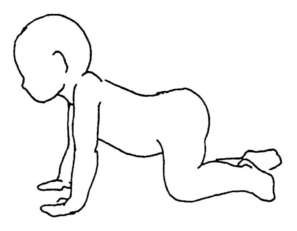

Exercise 20: Turtle Tuck

Roll body into tight ball, supported on knees.

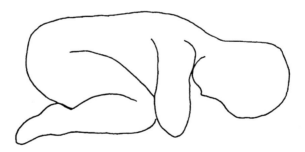

Exercise 21: Prone Extend and Arch

Alternate extension and back arch to turtle position.

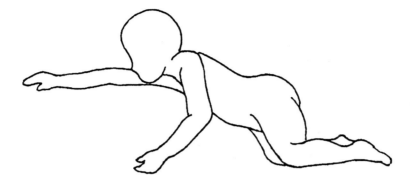

Exercise 22: Snake Crawl

Pull forward on stomach and "slither" along floor or mat like a snake.

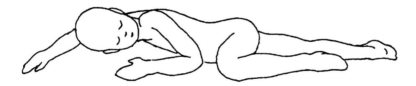

Exercise 23: Circular Prone Pivot

Twist and rotate on stomach in circular direction.

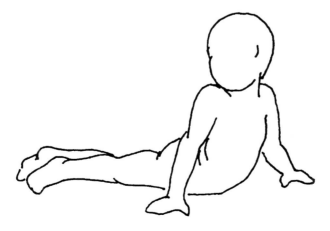

Exercise 24: One-hand Prone Push

Push-up with one arm to rotate trunk slightly to the side.

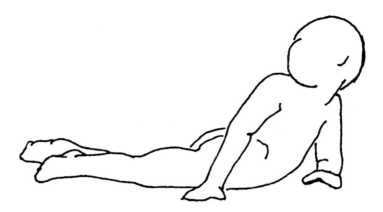

Exercise 25: Prone Swim

Lift arms over head one at a time in swimming motion forward.

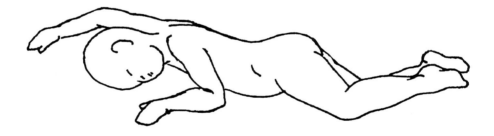

Exercise 26: Prone Walk-up

Pattern child to push up on elbows and "walk-up" to arms with feet.

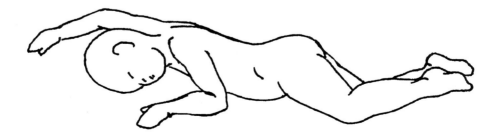

Exercise 27: Prone Crawl Down Incline

Child pulls forward on stomach utilizing the pull of gravity to move down a large incline mat.

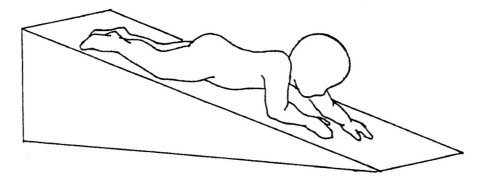

Exercise 28: Prone Crawl Up Incline

Child pulls forward on stomach up a large incline mat.

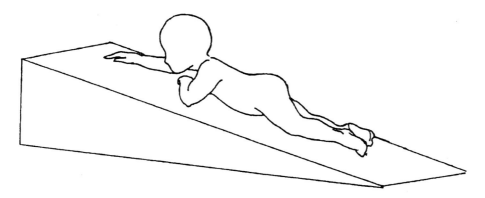

Exercise 29: Scooter Pull

Lay child on scooter-board. Encourage child to extend the arm using distal reach. Pull to move forward.

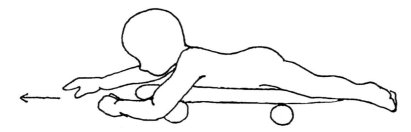

Exercise 30: Scooter Push

Guide the child through movements to push backwards on scooter-board.

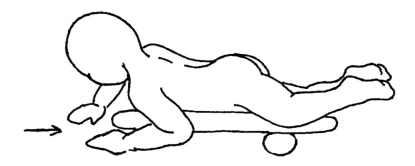

Rolling Position

Movements will be from supine to prone, prone to supine, and rolling over using different equipment.

Motion Control:	All body parts are used following specific directions.
Muscle Groups:	All muscle groups are utilized through rolling movements increasing trunk strength, control, and providing vestibular stimulation.

Exercise 31: Log Roll Right

Stretch arms over head and hold toy. Roll from supine to side position and side to supine (see Figure 7.6).

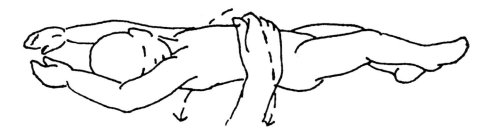

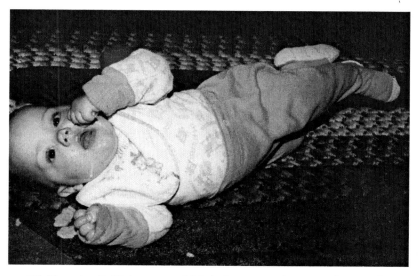

Figure 7.6. Exercise 5: This young girl is being assisted in completing a knee pat.

Exercise 32: Log Roll Left

Stretch arms over head holding an object. Roll to the left, supine to side and side to supine.

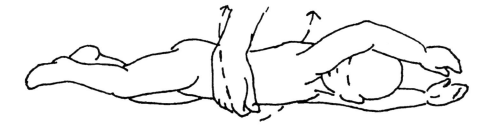

Exercise 33: Roll Over Rover

Roll supine to prone and prone to supine.

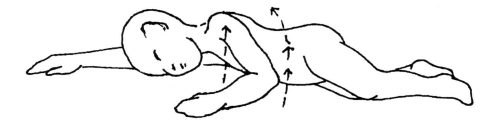

Exercise 34: Roll and Knee Touch

Roll to side. Flex one leg. Lift flexed leg over and touch knee to mat.

Exercise 35: Roll Down Incline Mat

Place child on large incline mat. Place your hands on the child's shoulder and hip. Using gravity, assist child with rolling down mat.

Exercise 36: Roll Up Incline Mat

Assist child with rolling up the mat by placing your hands on the child's shoulder and hip.

Exercise 37: Rolling Slowly

Place child on soft 8"–10" mat and encourage her to roll supine to prone very slowly while looking at visual target.

Exercise 38: Speed Rolling

Roll quickly down an incline mat, across a soft, thick mat, then across the room to knock down plastic objects (e.g., bowling pins).

Exercise 39: Blanket Roll

Roll up in soft blanket or sheet and then unroll.

Exercise 40: Bubble Roll

Log roll through a space of many blown bubbles floating in the air.

Four-Point Creeping

A normal creeping position should easily be maintained against the pull of gravity demonstrating good head control and upper-extremity support. Give guided support and patterning of movements as necessary to assist with specific exercises.

Motion Control: All body parts are used while performing specific movements.

Muscle Groups: All muscle groups are strengthened with repetitions to facilitate motor control and balance.

Exercise 41: Elbow-Knee Support

Provide support to child to help child maintain weight on elbows and knees.

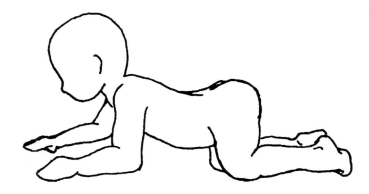

Exercise 42: Lift-up

Lift child's head up and down while child maintains support on elbows and knees. Encourage child to lift head up and down (without your support) while visually tracking a toy.

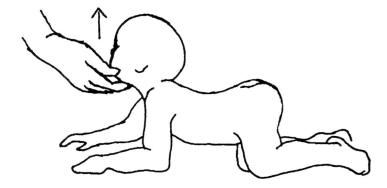

Exercise 43: 4-pt. Progression

Support in 4-pt. position on hands and knees. Turn head side to side and move up and down. Provide support under stomach and at hips to maintain position. Observe noticeable muscle tone changes in position of arms or legs.

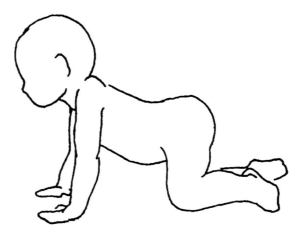

Exercise 44: Rocker

Gently rock the child forward and backward to establish rhythmical stabilization and increase strength.

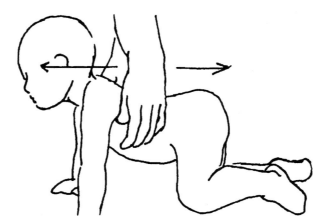

Exercise 45: Monkey Crawl

Move arm and leg forward on the same side of body (homolateral) for a specific distance.

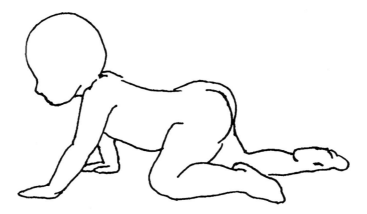

Exercise 46: Cross-lateral Creep

Creep forward using the arm and leg of the opposite side of the body.

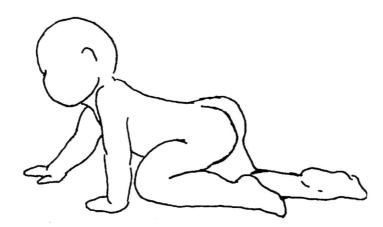

Exercise 47: Head-up Creep

Provide a visual target/toy raised slightly above the child's head and ask him/her to creep forward while looking at target/toy.

Exercise 48: Directionality Creep

Assist the child with moving forward, backward, and sideward while maintaining the 4-pt. creeping position.

Exercise 49: Down-hill Creep

Creep down an incline mat while focusing on a target.

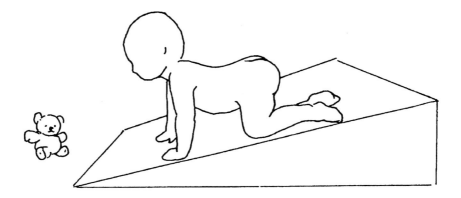

Exercise 50: Up-hill Creep

Creep up an incline mat while maintaining balance.

Exercise 51: Over the Hill

Arrange mats to create a "hilly" crawling/creeping course. Challenge the child by increasing the distance and height of the sequence of hills.

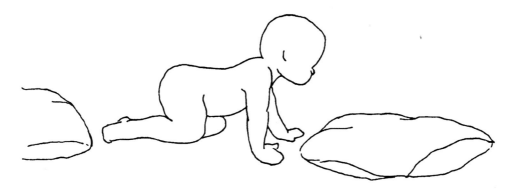

Exercise 52: Under the Table

Arrange several obstacles that the child must lower himself/herself to move under.

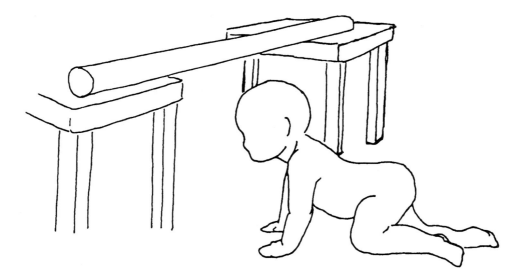

Exercise 53: Kick-Back and Up

Child assumes 4-pt. position. Assist child to extend one leg back and up. Support extended leg slightly at thigh, allowing child to maintain balance in 4-pt. position. Repeat with the other leg.

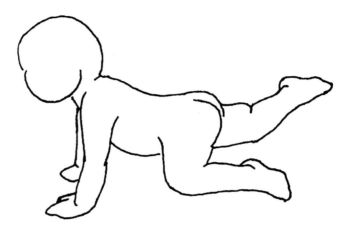

Exercise 54: Creeping with Weights

Place 1/4 lb. to 1/2 lb. ankle weights on the child. Have the child creep around play area.

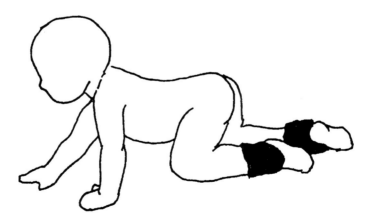

Exercises for Progression to Standing and Locomotion

This series of exercises moves from sitting position, kneeling, pulling/pushing up to standing and stepping patterns of locomotion. All exercises will assist with increasing muscle tone, strength, motor control, and balance. As stressed with previous positioning and patterning exercises, specificity of skill is dependent on the development of muscle tone and strength in all muscle groups.

Exercise 55: Knee Balance

Rise from 4-pt. creeping position to kneeling. Provide support at hips and under arms to help maintain balance.

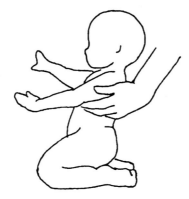

Exercise 56: Directional Kneeling

While maintaining kneeling position, assist the child with leaning from side to side while holding his/her head erect.

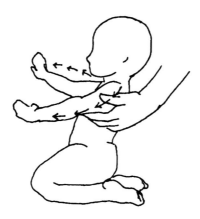

Exercise 57: Knee Walking

Assist the child with walking forward on knees and moving backward on knees. Hips should be lifted during forward progression.

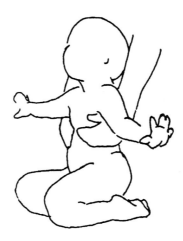

Exercise 58: Resisting Push

Assist the child with pushing against an object while maintaining balance. Push the child gently to the side and forward while providing support as needed.

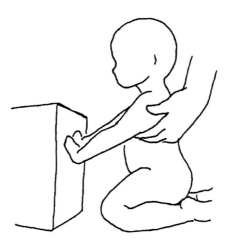

Exercise 59: Single Knee Balance

Raise one knee and place foot flat on floor while balancing on other knee. Provide assistance as needed for balance.

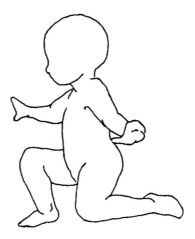

Exercise 60: Pull and Push to Stand

Guide child to pull-up to standing placing arms on a support while pushing up from one foot. Provide equal time for practicing rising to stand from other foot with continuous up and down motion. Provide assistance to maintain balance.

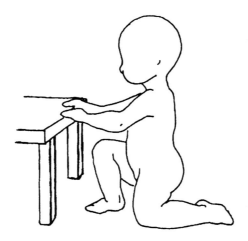

Exercise 61: Parallel Bar Stepping

Support by low (e.g., 18") pediatric parallel bars, facilitate the child through a stepping action by lifting and placing his/her foot forward.

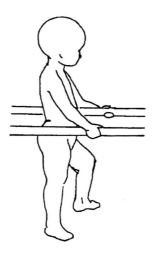

Exercise 62: Backward Stepping

Walk backwards using parallel bars for support.

Exercise 63: Sideward Stepping

Slide hands along parallel bars while stepping sideward.

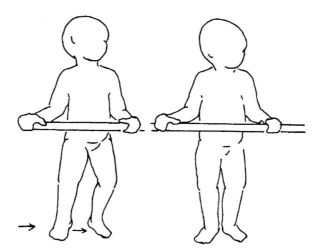

Exercise 64: Parallel Bar Stepping with Weights

Use 1/4 lb. and 1/2 lb. ankle weights to provide light resistance. Facilitate the child through a stepping action back and forth the distance of the parallel bars. Record the distance walked or number of sequences, repetitions, and sets (see Figure 7.7).

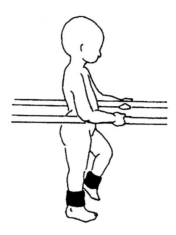

Exercise 65: Standing Knee Lifts

Supported by the side of the parallel bar, lift the knee up and down to develop upper leg and hip strength. Repeat with other knee/leg. As strength increases, provide light resistance with ankle weights. Record sequences, repetitions, and sets for progressive training.

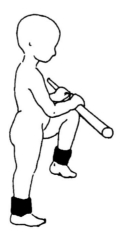

Exercise 66: Side Leg Lifts

Using the parallel bar for support, lift leg to the side allowing for strengthening of abductor and adductor muscles.

Exercise 67: Stair Stepping

Using 4"–6" step, assist the child with stepping up and down while using the railing for support.

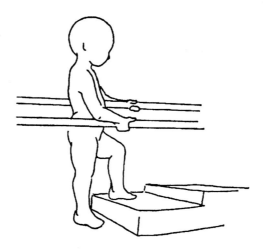

Exercise 68: Side Leg Circles

Lift leg to side and perform leg circles, forward and backward.

Exercise 69: Stepping Over Obstacles

Supported by parallel bars, assist the child with walking forward and stepping over low obstacles placed in pathway. Follow the same sequence with the child wearing light ankle weights for resistance.

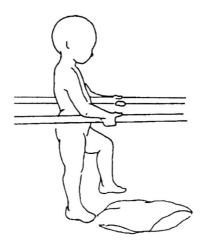

ENHANCING THE EXERCISES

Most of the exercises will be completed with a professional or parent working with a single individual. The exercises can be made more fun or play-like, by the adult singing simple children's songs or by the addition of small equipment (balloons, bubbles, bean bags, favorite toys, etc.). The adult can hold the object or place it on the floor, while encouraging the child to focus on it. Once a child has reached the capability of creeping or walking, then partner and small group instruction is more feasible. The following activities are provided as a foundation and can be further expanded in accord with the motivation and creativity of the adult. In reality however, the type of activities developed are also limited by the space, equipment, and personnel available.

Exercise 35: With 2 mats, who can be the first to roll down and knock over a bowling pin?

Exercise 44: Place a bean bag, toy, or scarf on the back of each child. How quickly can the child rock back and forth to have the object land on the floor?

Exercise 49 and 50: Who can reach the top or bottom of the incline mat to grasp a toy or touch the teacher's hand? Who can reach the top or bottom of the mat by the time the teacher finishes singing a song? Place a scarf over the child and have her move up or down the mat to uncover herself.

Exercise 51 and 52: Create an obstacle course with pillows, a small mat covering tire inner-tubes, a tunnel, 2 chairs with a rope across them to go under, very low objects to go over (poly spots, rope, cloth), geometric forms to crawl through, and so forth. The course can be followed with weights on the child's ankles (exercise 54) or it can be followed with the child moving in a kneeling position (exercise 57).

Exercise 53: Kick to touch a hanging object (balloon, ball, bubbles).

Exercise 58: With a partner, place a large ball in between the 2 children, and have them push toward each other.

Exercises 61–67: Walk toward a partner (child or mother) and touch that person, march to music, sing silly songs or chant a rhyme and have the child develop a rhythm as he walks, have the child move to get a special toy (see Figure 7.7).

If a group of children are older and have increased language or cognitive levels, game-like situations can be developed. Peer buddies or peer tutors can be very effective in assisting young children and increase the enjoyment of the activity for the children. Depending on the number of adults or peers that are available to assist the teacher, increased pieces of adaptive equipment may be needed to position the children. The type of positioning equipment that is utilized depends on the individual needs of each child. Working with a physical and/or occupational therapist will assist in determining the adaptive equip-

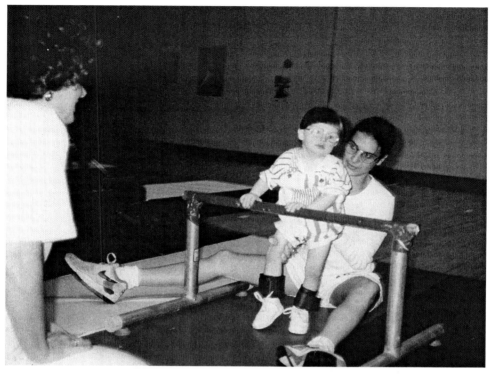

Figure 7.7. Exercise 64: Ankle weights increase leg strength as the movement specialist assists the child in standing and lifting his leg.

ment that is needed. Maintaining the position in which the child is placed for increasing time periods results in increasing the muscle tone. Simple finger plays (e.g., ten little indians), large body puzzles, balloon and bubble activities, and ball activities can be incorporated into the lesson to increase child engagement and fun.

REFERENCES

Brown, S. L., & Donovan, C. M. (1981). *Stimulation activities.* Ann Arbor: University of Michigan.

Brown, S., & Donovan, C. (1989). *Developmental programming for infants and young children—5 volumes.* Ann Arbor: University of Michigan.

Bricker, D., & Waddell, M. (2002). *Assessment, evaluation, and programming system: Curriculum for birth to three year, Vol. 3.* Baltimore: Brookes.

Eichstaedt, C. B., & Kalakian, L. H. (1993). *Developmental/Adapted physical activity: Making ability count.* New York: Macmillan.

Fisher, A. G., Murray, E. A., & Bundy, A. C. (1991). *Sensory integration theory and practice.* Philadelphia: F. A. Davis.

Frankenburg, W. K., Dodds, J., Archer, P., Bresnick, B., Maschka, P., Edelman, N., & Shapiro, H. (1992). *Denver II.* Denver, CO: Denver Developmental Materials.

Furuno, S., O'Reilly, K. A., Hosaka, C. M., Inatsuka, T. T., Allman, T. L., & Zeisloft, B. (2005). *HELP: Hawaii early learning profile and activity guide.* Palto Alto, CA: VORT.

Getman, G. N., Kane, E. R., Haigren, M. R., & McKee, G. W. (1968). *Developing learning readiness.* St. Louis: McGraw Hill.

Johnson-Martin, N. M., Jens, K. G., Attermeier, S. M., & Hacker, B. J. (1990). *The Carolina curriculum for preschoolers with special needs.* Baltimore: Paul H. Brookes.

Johnson-Martin, N. M., Jens, K. G., Attermeier, S. M., & Hacker, B. J. (1991). *The Carolina curriculum for infants and toddlers with special needs.* Baltimore: Paul H. Brookes.

Kephart, N. C. (1962). *The slow learner in the classroom.* Columbus, OH: Charles E. Merrill.

Knott, M., & Voss, D. E. (1968). *Proprioceptive neuromuscular facilitation.* New York: Harper & Row.

McCulloch, L. (1983). *A handbook for developing perceptual-motor and sensory skills through body movement.* Austin, TX: Tracor.

Montgomery, P., & Richter, E. (1978). *Sensorimotor integration for developmentally disabled children.* Los Angeles: Western Psychological Services.

Parks, S. (Ed.) (2004). *HELP strands: Curriculum-based developmental assessment birth to three years.* Palo Alto, CA: VORT.

Parks, S. (2006). *Inside HELP: Administration and reference manual.* Palo Alto, CA:VORT.

Rosato, F. D. (1990). *Fitness and wellness.* St. Paul, MN: West.

Sherrill, C. (2004). *Adapted physical activity, recreation and sport: Crossdisciplinary and lifespan* (6th ed.). New York: McGraw Hill.

Valett, R. E. (1967). *The remediation of learning disability.* Palo Alto, CA: Fearon.

Williamson, G. G. (1987). *Children with spina bifida: Early intervention and programming.* Baltimore: Paul H. Brookes.

Chapter 8

ACTIVITIES FOR REFLEX INTEGRATION AND DECREASING MUSCLE TONE

Chapter Objectives: After studying this chapter, the reader will be able to:
1. Discuss the organization of space, scheduling, and environmental factors in providing intervention services to young children with atypical muscle tone, lack of reflex integration, sensory motor delays, and manipulative problems (see Chapters 7, 8, 9, 10);
2. Give a description for assessment procedures of each tonic neck reflex and describe why the reflex may cause delay of development of specific motor milestones;
3. Design an individualized exercise program for a young child for integration of identified reflexes and to decrease muscle tone.
4. Develop a program of relaxation exercise for young children with hypertonicity.
5. Introduce therapeutic riding as a program to decrease hypertonicity and develop equilibrium/balance.

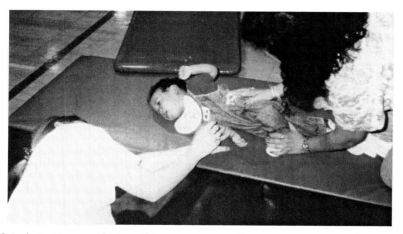

Figure 8.1. Activities are designed to encourage reflex integration and decrease hypertonicity.

263

Muscle tone provides the foundation for movement and allows any individual to be "ready" to perform simple motor actions. It is regulated by the cerebellar region of the brain and cannot be voluntarily controlled by the individual. Increased or exaggerated muscle tone (hypertonicity) is detrimental to voluntary movement and may be an "indicator" of primitive reflexes. Primitive reflexes are integrated as the child's central nervous system matures during the first year of life. Their existence hinders the development of independent movement, and after age 7 years, interferes with spatial and kinesthetic skills needed for academics. When primitive reflexes are present, the child is unable to progress to more advanced movement patterns and skills (see Chapters 3 and 5).

The purpose of the following activities is to decrease delayed neurological actions (i.e., primitive reflexes) that cause increased muscle tone or hypertonicity and interfere with obtaining functional movement skills (e.g., rolling, creeping). The following assessment procedures should be considered: (a) assess for presence of reflexes which would indicate delayed motor development; (b) assess functional movement skills to determine motor delays or patterns that exist due to presence of abnormal reflex patterns; and (c) demonstrate correct positioning and handling to prevent inappropriate sensory excitation that would cause strengthening of primitive reflex patterns.

ASSESSMENT OF ASYMMETICAL TONIC NECK REFLEX
(0 to 4–6 MOS.)

Supine Position

Turning of the head to the side causes extension of the arm on the face side and flexion of the arm at the back of the head.

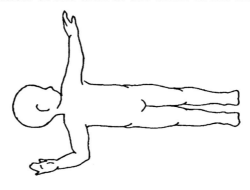

Motion Control: Interferes with rolling over, voluntary hand positioning, reaching, and midline skills.

ACTIVITIES FOR INTEGRATION OF ASYMMETRICAL TONIC NECK REFLEX

Supine Position–On back, arms at sides, palms of hands down, legs extended–is used in several activities.

Activity 1: Head-Neck Synchronizer

Turn head from side to side while maintaining position with palms flat on mat and:
- Touch ears to the floor
- Look in mirror at face
- Name pictures/colors on wall
- When turning head to the right, touch nose with the right hand.

Activity 2: Extremity Twiddle

- Lift arms and reach for the sky while passing favorite toy from one hand to the other (see figure below).
- Raise hand to touch lifted bent knee on same side of body, then on other side of body.
- Move extended arms above head with head remaining flat on mat; move legs out from midline with arms and return to starting position.
- Turn head from side to side while flexing arms to touch shoulders.

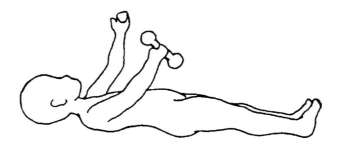

Activity 3: Rolling Sequences

- Move arms and legs to flexed, tucked position and rock from side to side then back and forth.
- With one hand on child's hips and other hand on child's shoulder, roll child over slowly to side and back to supine position.
- Assist child with rolling completely over while keeping hands at sides.
- Extend the arms above the child's head and place toy in hands and assist child with performing log roll to the left and then to the right.
- Roll down incline mat.
- Roll up incline mat.

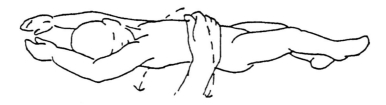

Activity 4: Four-Point Movements

- Support child in 4-pt. position while rocking side to side and back and forth.
- Creep forward, backward, and side to side.
- Have child lift head and look at target placed forward and slightly above head level then look down at floor target. Repeat.
- Creep up and down an incline

ASSESSMENT OF TONIC LABYRINTHINE SUPINE REFLEX (0 TO 4–6 MOS.)

In back lying position the child demonstrates increasee extensor tone of the extremities.

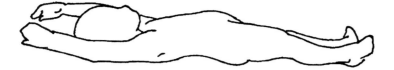

Motion Control: Interferes with raising of the head, bending of knees, reaching for feet, and bringing of hands to midline.

ACTIVITIES FOR INTEGRATION OF TONIC LABYRINTHINE SUPINE REFLEX

Supine Position–On back, arms at sides, palms of hands down, legs flat on mat–is used in several activities.

Activity 5: Head-toe Flexion Activities

- Lift head, touch chin to chest and look at knees.
- Extend legs and flex toes to chest.
- Lift head to chest while looking at flexed toes (see figure below).
- Lie on side and bend the head while flexing knees and toes.

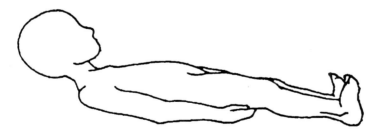

Activity 6: Tight Tuck Series

- Flex arms across chest and touch the knees to arms.
- Raise head and chest upward to knees (bent-knee sit-up); support under head/trunk as needed with incline mat.
- While in tight tuck position rock back and forth.
- While in tight tuck position egg roll from side to side.

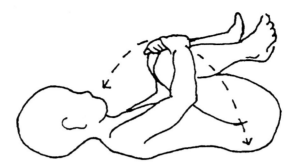

Activity 7: Rolling Sequence Activities

- With arms flexed across chest log roll slowly, then quickly.
- With arms flexed or extended log roll down incline mat.
- Roll to side; lift flexed knee over body and touch mat (see figure below).
- Wrap in blanket and roll slowly side to side and supine to prone to supine.

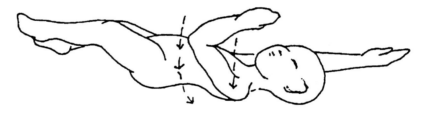

Activity 8: Visual and Tactile Stimulation Activities

Using small (i.e., 2"–3") suspended ball, perform the following activities:

- Suspend ball over the feet and tap gently with each foot while touching chin to chest and looking at ball.
- Suspend ball over chest and tap ball gently back and forth using both hands.
- Suspend ball over child's face and encourage him/her to visually track ball from side to side.
- Suspend the ball at child's waist. Flex the child's body to tuck position and encourage him/her to touch ball with elbows and knees.

ASSESSMENT OF TONIC LABYRINTHINE PRONE RELEX
(0 to 4–6 MOS.)

Prone position—when lying on the stomach the child demonstrates increased flexion.

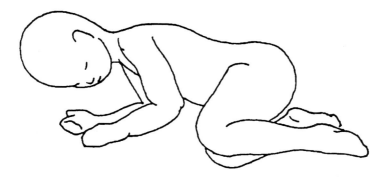

Motion Control: Interferes with lifting of head, extension of arms and legs, and distal reaching.

ACTIVITIES FOR INTEGRATION OF TONIC LABYRINTHINE PRONE REFLEX

Prone position—on stomach, arms extended over head, legs extended—is the starting position for many of the following activities.

Activity 9: Head Rotation and Lift Activities

- Lift (extend) head and neck and focus on toy or target.
- Raise arms and abduct to each side.
- Provide support under child's chest with bolster. Have child reach across midline to grasp toy (right then left hand).
- Lift and rotate head to one side and look at toy by extended arm (shoulder level).

Activity 10: Airplane Extended Position Activities

- Lift arms and legs upward in extended position while arching back. Repeat.
- Rock back and forth in extended position.

- Roll side to side in extended position.
- Crawl forward with overarm swimming motion (see below).

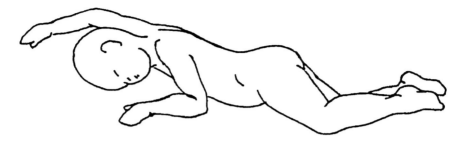

Activity 11: Scooter Board Activities

(Carpet squares can be substituted for some activities)
Using scooter board, perform the following exercises with the scooter board under the child's trunk and the child's arms and legs extended completely:

- Pull forward on scooter board while lifting legs from floor (see figure below).
- Push backward; spin around; change directions and repeat.
- Have child move around throughout individually designed obstacle course.

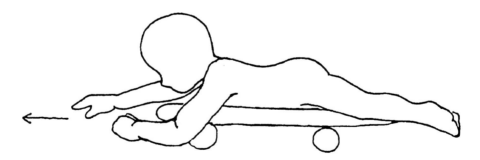

Activity 12: Proprioceptive-Vestibular-Visual Stimulation Activities

- Position on vestibular/rocking board in prone position rocking forward and backward while visually focusing on wall target.

- Rock side to side with arms and legs extended in airplane position.
- Roll child slowly from prone to side, and side to prone while tilting vestibular board in opposite direction.
- Place child in 4-pt. creeping position on rocking board and encourage child to maintain eye focus on wall.

ASSESSMENT OF SYMMETRICAL TONIC NECK REFLEX (0 to 6–8 MOS.)

Flexion of head causes flexion of the arms and extension of the legs; raising of the head causes arm extension and leg flexion (i.e., bunny-hop).

Motion Control: Interferes with creeping.

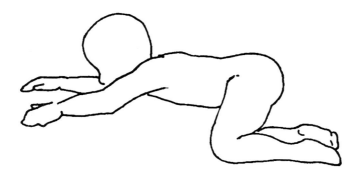

ACTIVITIES FOR INTEGRATION OF SYMMETRICAL TONIC NECK REFLEX

Activity 13: 4-pt. Creeping Activities

- Lift head up and down while keeping arms extended and legs flexed.
- Rotate head side to side while maintaining the position.
- Lift and reach up with one arm then the other while maintaining balance.
- Lift and extend one leg then the other while maintaining

balance (see figure below).
- Crawl/Creep forward, backward, sideward while maintaining visual focus on wall target.
- Bear crawl, crosslateral crawl, seal-crawl.
- Inchworm reach forward and backward.
- Maintain 3-point balance and reach/extend arm across the midline to pick up toy.
- Visually track a rolled ball or swinging ball from side to side.
- Perform mule kicks (kicking both legs up and back at the same time).

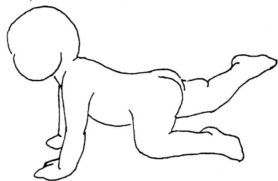

RELAXATION ACTIVITIES

Relaxation activities are essential to decreasing muscle tone and to facilitate movement. The following are suggested for individuals at any age and at various functioning levels.

- Rhythmic massage
- Use warm towels for rubbing arms/legs to increase circulation
- Soft instrumental music
- Deep and slow breathing exercises
- Soft/low lighted environment
- Stretch and melt exercises
- Cool-down activities
- Tactile stimulation with vibrators

- Aquatic therapy/whirlpools
- Imagery: rag dolls, ice cream, snow melting, moving in a jar of syrup, fluffy clouds floating in the sky, a furry puppy sleeping, bubbles blown in air, slowly running water, snowflakes falling, sifting sand, sailing boats
- Swinging, swaying, stretching, and bending activities

ENHANCING THE ACTIVITIES

Each of the preceding activities provides examples to modify and enrich the exercises to facilitate integration of reflexes. As the motor functioning level of a child increases, and partner or small group activities are involved in intervention, the motor specialist could consider the following:

- Incorporating warm-up movement routines prior to skill activities,
- Inclusion of flexibility movements to prevent increased tension,
- Proper positioning to prevent primitive reflex patterns from becoming stimulated,
- Appropriate positioning to allow for maximum participation in motor and other daily class activities through the use of adaptive equipment,
- Specific motor/play activities designed to prevent the child from maintaining the same position/posture for long time periods.

THERAPEUTIC RIDING

A well-planned therapeutic riding program is extremely beneficial for relaxing muscle tone in children with disabilities. It can also increase strength for children who demonstrate hypotonic development and have a visibly calming affect on children who tend to be hyperactive. Therefore, children with spina bifida, cerebral palsy, autism, Down syndrome, mental retardation, muscular dystrophy, visual impairments, and other developmental delays, will benefit from therapeutic riding. The children respond to the horses as if they were extra-large teddy bears made for hugging!

During a therapeutic riding session, 5–6 children are each on their own horse. Each child is assisted up a ramp to mount the horse. Once on the horse, a volunteer walker on each side of the horse assists in stabilization of the child, while another volunteer is leading the horse. The child is told to sit up straight maintaining posture, look between the horse's ears, loosely hold the reins, keep feet in stirrups and post if possible, while the horse is walking. Children are challenged to maintain balance while horses move forward around the arena, stop, turn, reverse the direction in which they are moving, and step over low obstacles. When the arena director instructs the horses to move to the middle of the arena, children are requested to touch parts of the horse (i.e., tail, ears), turn to the back of the saddle, and touch parts of their body. All of these skills require maintenance of balance and equilibrium, and provide practice with body part identification, laterality and directionality (see Figure 8.2).

Socialization is a valuable asset of therapeutic riding not only for the children, but for the entire family. Smiles and laughter are very apparent among parents as they visit and watch the children enjoying a structured series of riding routines. "Not only do they sit taller and smile more, they extend their dreams beyond the confines of their disability, into new, unexplored worlds. For individuals with impaired mobility, horseback riding gently and rhythmically moves their bodies in a manner similar to the human walking gait" (Hartzell,

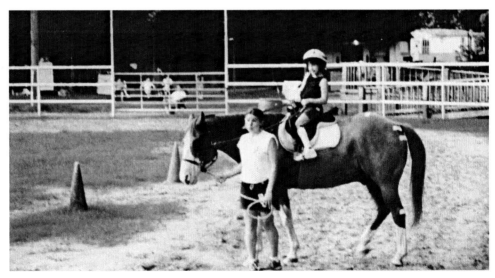

Figure 8.2. An adult leads the horse and provides directions, while the child maintains sitting balance and helps guide the horse throughout the lesson.

GNOTRC, New Orleans, Summer, 2005).

Children with various disabilities were followed through therapeutic riding activities to record changes in their motor capabilities. EB, a child with cerebral palsy was studied extensively at the University of New Orleans Pediatric Adapted Motor Development and Physical Education Clinic and at the Greater New Orleans Therapeutic Riding Center. The technique of kinetic analysis of movement was used to evaluate changes in EB after therapeutic riding. EB was premarked with tape on specific joints allowing for observation and photographic analysis of her posture, balance, muscle control, and strength. Prior to riding, the stride of EB's steps were measured by the use of vertical and horizontal grids. After a 30-minute riding lesson, her gait width of stepping stride for both left and right legs was measured by use of the grids. EB had increased in flexibility, range of motion, and length of stride in her stepping patterns (see Figures 8.3 and 8.4).

Several children with Down syndrome were observed over numerous occasions whereby their attention span extended past 20 minutes while following directions when riding. Children with learning disorders increased concentration, patience and discipline. The unique relationship formed between the rider and the horse is unexplainable; however, confidence and self esteem are greatly increased. Other activities that may be beneficial for the same children simply can not be compared to a therapeutic riding session.

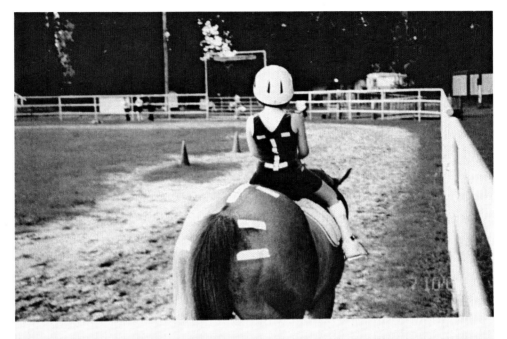

Figures 8.3 and 8.4. Both figures indicate the use of kinetic analysis of movement for this young child during therapeutic horseback riding.

REFERENCES

Brown, S. L., & Donovan, C. M. (1981). *Stimulation activities.* Ann Arbor: University of Michigan.

Brown, S., & Donovan, C. M. (1989). *Developmental programming for infants and young children–5 volumes.* Ann Arbor: University of Michigan.

Bricker, D., & Waddell, M. (2002). *Assessment, evaluation, and programming system: Curriculum for birth to three years.* Baltimore: Brookes.

Eichstaedt, C. B., & Kalakian, L. H. (1993). *Developmental/Adapted physical activity: Making ability count.* New York: MacMillan.

Fisher, A. G., Murray, E. A., & Bundy, A. (1991). *Sensory integration theory and practice.* Philadelphia: F. A. Davis.

Frankenburg, W. K., Dodds., J., Archer, P., Bresnick, B., Maschka, P., Edelman, N., & Shapiro, H. (1992). *Denver II.* Denver, CO: Denver Developmental Materials.

Furuno, S., O'Reilly, K. A., Hosake, C. M., Inatsuka, T. T., Allman, T. L., & Zeisloft, B. (1985). *HELP activity guide.* Palto Alto, CA: VORT.

Getman, G. N., Kane, E. R., Halgren, M. R., & McKee, G. W. (1968). *Developing learning readiness.* St. Louis, MO: McGraw-Hill.

Johnson-Martin, N. M., Jens, K. G., Attermeier, S. M., & Hacker, B. J. (1990). *The Carolina curriculum for preschoolers with special needs.* Baltimore: Paul H. Brookes.

Kephart, N. C. (1962). *The slow learner in the classroom.* Columbus, OH: Charles E. Merrill.

Knott, M., & Voss, D. E. (1968). *Proprioceptive neuromuscular facilitation.* New York: Harper & Row.

McCulloch, L. (1983). *A handbook for developing perceptual-motor and sensory skills through body movement.* Austin, TX: Tracor.

Parks, S. (Ed.). (1992a). *HELP strands: Curriculum-based developmental assessment.* Palo Alto, CA: VORT.

Parks, S. (1992b). *Inside HELP.* Palo Alto, CA: VORT.

Rosato, F. D. (1990). *Fitness and wellness.* St. Paul, MN: West.

Sherrill, C. (1993). *Adapted physical activity, recreation and sport: Crossdisciplinary and lifespan* (4th ed.). Dubuque, IA: Brown & Benchmark.

Valett, R. E. (1967). *The remediation of learning disability.* Palo Alto, CA: Fearon.

Williamson, G. G. (1987). *Children with spina bifida: Early intervention and programming.* Baltimore: Paul H. Brookes.

Chapter 9

ACTIVITIES FOR SENSORY MOTOR DEVELOPMENT

Chapter Objectives: After studying this chapter, the reader will be able to:
1. Identify the role of sensory modalities in relation to movement problems of young children;
2. Develop an additional motor development program for sensory motor stimulation, according to the child's strengths and weaknesses in each specific sensory modality.

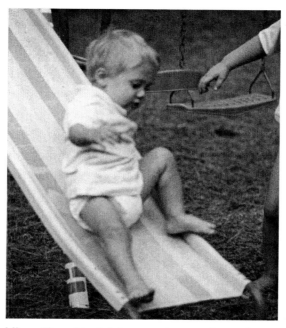

Figure 9.1. This toddler utilizes his righting reactions in descending a slide. This chapter presents activities for developing postural reactions and vestibular stimulation.

279

Sensory motor development is critical to the child's performance of movement patterns and motor skills. As input into the central nervous system, it provides the foundation for movement. When analyzing movement difficulties, it is important to identify the role of sensory modalities in relation to movement problems. Sensory motor input problems are responsible not only for the performance of elementary movement patterns, but may also influence higher level motor proficiency. The children in the following examples indicate inappropriate equilibrium responses: an infant who is unable to maintain alignment of head with body in a sitting position, and a preschool child who has difficulty and shows tension trying to perform a 1-foot balance. Both children indicate a sensory motor problem relating to the vestibular system and would benefit from vestibular intervention activities.

This chapter highlights activities for sensory motor development, including vestibular stimulation, visual motor control, auditory discrimination, and tactile stimulation. Each modality is specific and activities can be developed to highlight remediation of each modality. However, because the modalities may provide feedback to the central nervous system simultaneously, it may be difficult to isolate each modality during movement intervention. For example, when rocking on a vestibular ball, a child is being provided kinesthetic, vestibular, and tactile feedback, and by requesting the child to maintain gaze on the adult's face, the child is also required to maintain visual motor control.

ACTIVITIES FOR POSTURAL REACTIONS AND VESTIBULAR STIMULATION

Automatic responses to maintaining equilibrium and balance of the infant/toddler are termed postural reactions. They should be developed in young children by the age of 2–10 months and continue developing throughout the lifespan. Three categories compose reactions: (a) righting (head, neck, body), (b) parachute, and (c) equilibrium. Stimulation of the vestibular sensory modality develops balance and movement control. Assessment procedures should include: (a) assessment of reactions to see if the child has the necessary protective skills to prevent injury (i.e., attempts to catch self when losing balance or falling), and (b) assessment of functional movement skills to determine motor delays that exist due to poor balance skills. Activities will be presented in the following sequences: (a) righting reactions, (b) parachute and protective extension, and (c) equilibrium and balance.

1: Righting Reaction Activities

- Rolling exercises
- While providing some support in sitting position, move and tilt the child from side to side and front to back; allow the child to adjust and maintain sitting position.
- Using tilt or vestibular board, provide rocking stimulation in prone, supine, sitting, and 4-pt. positions.
- Using physioball/vestibular ball with child supported in prone position, rock ball side to side, forward and backward; repeat in sitting position.
- Place the child in prone position on scooter board and assist him/her with pushing forward, backward, side to side, or spinning.

2: Parachute Reaction-Protective Extension Activities

- Assist the child with performing swinging and swaying movements while supporting child in prone and sitting positions.
- Using physioball/vestibular ball place the child in prone position and rock forward and backward causing the child to reach-out in protective extension.
- Using vestibular board, repeat above listed activities.
- Perform scooter board activities listed above.

3: Equilibrium & Balance Activities (Total body responses)

- Rolling activities.
  -down & up inclines
  -through obstacle courses
  -at targets (e.g., bowling pins)
  -holding ball between feet
  -tuck rolling side to side, over, back/forth rocking.
- Vestibular board—rock in prone, supine, sitting and 4-point positions (see Figure 9.2).
- Physioball/vestibular ball—prone, supine, and sitting.
- Scooter board exercises—prone, supine, sitting, racing, obstacle

course.
- 4-point position balance exercises with visual targets and blindfold-ed, reaching for target or hanging mobile.
- Animal movements (e.g., bear crawl, measuring worm, seal crawl, elephant walk, rooster walk, frog jumping, mule kick).
- Walking patterns:
  -cross-lateral pattern: right arm and left leg forward, left arm and right leg forward.
  -following footprint patterns on floor
  -grapevine stepping pattern: step side with left, cross over in front with right, step side with left, cross behind leg with right, and continue pattern
  -stepping over obstacles
  -tire obstacle courses
  -backward walking
  -tip-toe and heel patterns
  -on heavily matted surface
  -up and down inclines
  -stepping through ladder rungs
  -walking between ropes, poles, crooked paths, taped lines, on ropes.
- Walking board/balance beam.
- Movements up/down stairs.
- Running through obstacles.
- Stopping, starting, changing directions, and dodging obstacles.
- Marching to music.
- Two-foot jumping activities: jump down, in and out, over; jump consecutively; jump for distance; jump forward, sideways, and backwards; jump over swinging rope.
- One-foot balance activities: on dominant foot, non-dominant foot, with and without assistance (holding onto rail or person); using different arm positions; balance with eyes blindfolded.

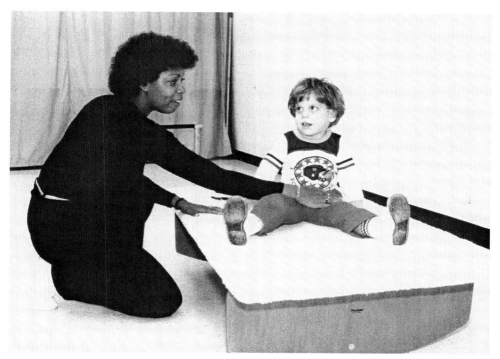

Figure 9.2. Activity 3: The child is being assisted to maintain sitting balance on a vestibular board.

ACTIVITIES FOR VISUAL MOTOR CONTROL

Visual motor control is defined as the ability to coordinate eye movements to fixate, track moving objects, discriminate between forms/objects, shapes, and sizes, and separate objects from the background. Exercises and activities are included for visual motor tracking and control, visual discrimination, and figure-ground perception. Assessment strategies should address the child's history for visual acuity (e.g., wearing of corrective lens), visual awareness and tracking skills, fine-motor grasp/release, form perception, and pencil/pen manipulation.

4: Visual Motor Tracking and Control Activities

• Child shows awareness of movements in surroundings.
• Child responds to changes in facial expressions of caregiver's face.
• Child visually tracks person or objects moving in room.

- Eyes respond to changes in light.
- Eyes track across midline from side to side, up and down, circular motion.
- Child visually attends to objects for 5–10 seconds.
- Child looks for hidden object.
- Child visually tracks a suspended ball.
- In supine, child raises head to look at wall target placed 12" from floor.
- In supine, child looks from wall to ceiling targets.
- In supine, child arches head/neck backward and looks from wall target to ceiling.
- Suspended ball exercises (e.g., ball can be suspended at any height, from eye level to feet):
  -sitting, track ball from side to side, up and down
  -kneeling, perform same
  -standing, perform same
  -reach out and touch swinging ball with forefinger, elbow, head, nose, foot, ear, etc.
  -touch left and right side body parts (hand, elbow, shoulder)
  -touch ball with front, back, sides, knee, foot.

Balloon activities: tap with one hand, tap with the other hand; tap with one finger; tap consecutively with each finger on the hand; tap with back of the hand, wrist, elbow; tap from one hand to the other; toss and catch; hit with one foot and the other foot.

- Mirror play and imitation of arm and leg movements, facial gestures, and simple finger plays.
- Ball bouncing exercises: bounce and catch, bounce consecutively, bounce to a target or partner, bounce high and low, bounce and walk.
- Place targets (e.g., forms-circle, square, triangle) on wall or on floor and have child swing the ball to hit target.
- Flashlight tracking activities side to side across midline, up and down, in patterns, around room, across ceiling.
- Ball rolling and tracking (see Figure 9.3).
- Beanbag tossing and throwing.
- Trace, imitate, and copy forms, letters, or numbers. Do these in sand; with whipping cream on any surface; on paper with crayons,

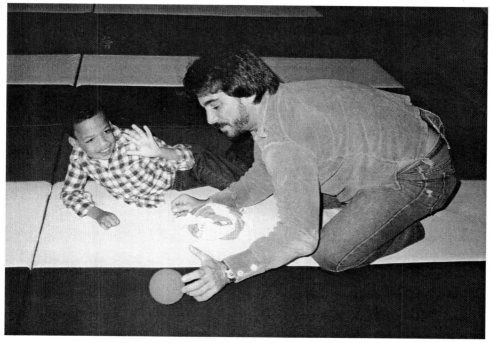

Figure 9.3. Activity 4: Visual tracking and control are required to engage in this ball activity.

pencil, or markers; painting with water on sidewalk; copying on a partner's back and have him/her guess form, number or letter.

5: Visual Motor Discrimination Activities

- Match shapes, colors, objects.
- Select objects of different shape and same shape.
- Blindfold child and have him/her identify shapes by feeling them.
- Child steps on shapes and identifies them by name.
- Call out name of shape and direct child to jump and hop on that shape.
- Design a grid pattern of lines in which child walks the outline of form patterns (square, triangle).
- Match and name shapes of objects; jump and call out name of objects; go through, over, under, around object that the care giver names; find, cut, and paste object that the caregiver names.
- Select large vs. small object; vary games with movements for size

discrimination.
• Make shapes with ropes.

6: Visual Figure-ground Perception Activities

• Overlapping geometric shapes.
  -walks on shapes in grid pattern
  -trace out shapes in maze
  -identify flashlight patterns designed on wall.
• Find and trace with hand objects hidden in drawings.
• Ball control activities.
  -bounce and catch a ball while focusing on wall target.
  -change from standing to kneeling while bouncing ball and focusing
   on target that caregiver names.
• Separate mixed letters to write name.
• Design obstacle courses in which child must move (e.g., crawl,
  creep, knee walk, walk, jump, hop, climb).

ACTIVITIES FOR AUDITORY DISCRIMINATION

This series of activities designed for children who are having difficulty discriminating between soft and loud sounds, high and low pitch-
es, responding to oral directions, and recalling information given in
sequences. Children who appear to have poor listening skills may
have problems with auditory discrimination; however, the child's history of hearing acuity examinations should be reviewed carefully.
Activities for auditory stimulation, auditory awareness, and auditory
discrimination are included below.

7: Auditory Discrimination Activities

• Responds to loud sounds (e.g., bells, hand claps).
• Vocalizes sounds (e.g., babbles, imitates sounds).
• Laughs and reacts to stimulation.
• Searches for sounds in room.
• Watches speaker's mouth, eyes.
• Imitates syllables/sounds.
• Responds to requests with sounds and gestures.
• Responds to name.

- Moves body to rhythm of music.
- Follows simple commands.
- Makes sounds to music.
- Matches sounds with example or picture of animal.
- Responds to directions (e.g., in, on, over, out, above, in front, behind).

8: Blindfold Activities

- Identify body part by touch.
- Place body in positions (e.g., back to wall, side to wall, hand on wall, foot on chair).
- Crawl, walk, and hop forward, backward and sideward.
- Clapping activities: one clap on stomach, two claps on knees, three claps to sit down.
- Log roll, egg roll, perform animal walks, etc.

9: Point of Balance Activities

- Call out positions and have the child assume position: foot and knee, two feet and one hand, both knees, one hand and knee on same side, opposite side; repeat.
- Do above on designated spot or carpet square.
- Balance with partner.

10: Angels in the Snow Activities (supine position)

- Move both arms along floor to shoulder level.
- Move both legs apart to "V" position.
- Move leg and arm on same side, then crosslateral, three body parts, and both arms and legs simultaneously.
- Perform same exercises blindfolded.

11: Listen and Imitate Activities (see Figure 9.4)

- Listen, count, and bounce ball same number of times.
- Bounce ball high with high pitch sound, low with low pitch sound.
- Be thin on high musical note, be small on low musical note.
- Tell time with body. Give child a time to put body in (i.e., 12 o'clock position, 9 o'clock position).

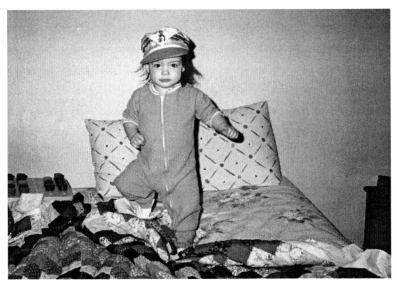

Figure 9.4. Activity 11: Child is imitating movement after listening to directions given by caregiver.

12: Sequencing Directions

- Start with one direction to follow, increase to two and eventually three.
- Step, sit, run.
- Toss, catch, and slide.
- Step/jump on sequence of forms, numbers, letters.

ACTIVITIES FOR TACTILE STIMULATION

The child's responses to tactile stimulation should be assessed for hypersensitivity or lack of reactions. Activities that follow are for increasing tactile awareness and decreasing sensitivity.

13: Tactile Stimulation Activities

- Touch and stroke the child's arms and legs to promote relaxation. Touch different body parts and ask child to call out parts.
- Use different textured fabrics (e.g., terry cloth, velvet, cotton) to stroke the child's arms and legs.

- Use different levels of tactile pressure (e.g., light, soft, firm, stroking, tickling, vibrator, and massage).
- Wrap colored tape around child's wrists and ankles. Ask child to touch body part with specific color of tape.
- Blindfold child and have him crawl on and through different surfaces/objects while naming them (e.g., form/shape box, rope lines, balance boards, scooter boards).
- Reach in box and identify objects by picking up and feeling them.
- Walk through obstacle course on different textured mats, carpet squares, water, sand, clay, etc.
- Angels-in-the-Snow Position (blindfolded).
- Perform various bilateral and cross lateral movements by caregiver naming or touching body part to be moved.

ACTIVITIES FOR KINESTHETIC AND SPATIAL AWARENESS

The kinesthetic modality provides sensory information from the muscles, tendons, and joints of the body and provides a means for communicating about position in space. Kinesthetic awareness is sometimes referred to as body or spatial awareness.

14: Body Positioning Activities

- Move body parts touched by caregiver.
- In supine position, move body parts by verbal directions (e.g., in, out, up, down).
- In prone position, move in and out of airplane position lifting head, arms, and legs upward.

15: Mirror Play

- Touch body parts while looking in mirror.
- Touch adult or partner body parts on command.
- Imitate caregiver's movements while looking in mirror.

16: Obstacle Course Play

- Perform different movement patterns (e.g., crawl, creep, roll) under, over, and through an obstacle course (see Figure 9.5).
- Walk forward and backward through obstacle course.

- Maneuver though specific obstacle course design on scooter boards and in different positions.

17: *Moving Shapes Activities*

- Have the child assume various shapes on soft mat (e.g., circle, tuck, letters, form) in prone then supine position.
- Swing, sway, stretch, twist, and bend the body.
- Using carpet squares do an arm pull, leg push, knee pull, carpet push, prone and supine bilateral and cross lateral arm/leg movements.
- In prone on scooter board pull, push, spin.
- Sitting on scooter board, push and pull an object.

18: *Balance Beam Activities* (provide support as needed, at hips or by holding hand)

- Walk forward, sideways, backwards.
- Maintain a balance position.
- Carry an object while walking on beam.
- Walk with beanbag on head or other body parts.
- Walk and step over objects or through hoop.

19: *Hula Hoop Directionality Activities*

- Sit in hula hoop and identify circular space.
- Step in, step out, jump over, jump in, jump out of hoop, crawl through hoop.
- Walk on hoop in a circle, walk backward, walk sideward.
- Do the above activities with a partner.
- Roll hoop and walk.
- Roll hoop to adult or partner.
- Swing hoop on 1 arm and then other arm.

20: *Animal Stunts*

- Elephant walk, seal crawl, egg roll, mule kick, bunny hop, inchworm.

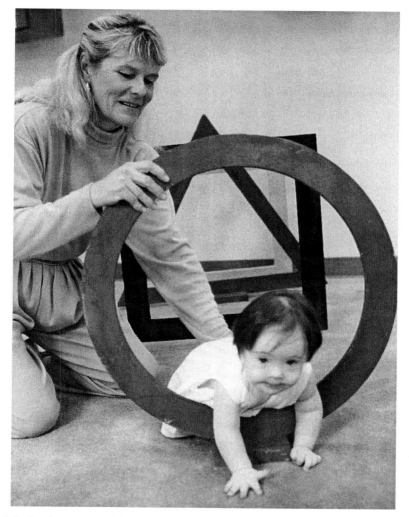

Figure 9.5. As the young child moves through shapes, she is demonstrating kinesthetic and spatial awareness.

REFERENCES

Bricker, D., & Waddell, M. (2002). *Assessment, evaluation and programming system: Curriculum for birth to three years, Vol. 3.* Baltimore: Brookes.

Brown, S. L. & Donovan, C. M. (1981). *Stimulation activities.* Ann Arbor: University of Michigan.

Brown, S., & Donovan, C. (1989). *Developmental programming for infants and young children—5 volumes.* Ann Arbor: University of Michigan.

Fisher, A. G., Murray, E. A., & Bundy, A. C. (2002). *Sensory integration theory and prac-*

tice (2nd ed.). Philadelphia: F. A..Davis.

Frankenburg, W. K., Dodds, J., Archer, P., Bresnick, B., Maschka, P., Edelman, N., & Shapiro, H., (1992). *Denver II.* Denver, CO: Denver Developmental Materials.

Furuno, S., O'Reilly, K. A., Hosaka, C. M., Inatsuka, T. T., Allman, T. L., & Zeisloft, B. (2005). *HELP activity guide.* Palo Alto, CA: VORT.

Getman, G. N., Kane, E. R., Halgren, M. R, & McKee, G. W. (1968). *Developing learning readiness.* St. Louis: McGraw-Hill.

Horvat, M., & Eichstaedt, C. B., (2003). *Developmental/Adapted physical activity: Making ability count* (4th ed.). San Francisco, CA: Benjamin Cummings.

Johnson-Martin, N. M., Jens, K. G., Attermeier, S. M., & Hacker, B. J. (1990). *The Carolina curriculum for preschoolers with special needs.* Baltimore: Brookes.

Johnson-Martin, N. M., Jens, K. G., Attermeier, S. M., & Hacker, B. (1991). *The Carolina curriculum for infants and toddlers with special needs.* Baltimore: Paul H. Brookes.

Kephart, N. C. (1962). *The slow learner in the classroom.* Columbus, OH: Charles E. Merrill.

Knott, M., & Voss, D. E. (1968). *Proprioceptive neuromuscular facilitation.* New York: Harper & Row.

McCulloch, L. (1983). *A handbook for developing perceptual motor and sensory skills through body movement.* Austin, TX: Tracor.

Montgomery, P., & Richter, E. (1978). *Sensorimotor integration for developmentally disabled children.* Los Angeles: Western Psychological Services.

Parks, S. (Ed.). (2004). *HELP strands: Curriculum-based developmental assessment.* Palo Alto, CA: VORT.

Parks, S. (2006). *Inside HELP: Administration and reference manual.* Palo Alto, CA: VORT.

Rosato, F. D. (1990). *Fitness and wellness.* St. Paul, MN: West.

Sherrill, C. (2004) *Adapted physical activity, recreation and sport: Crossdisciplinary and lifespan* (6th ed.). Boston: McGraw-Hill.

Valett, R. E. (1967). *The remediation of learning disability.* Palo Alto, CA: Fearon.

Williamson, G. G. (1987). *Children with spina bifida: Early intervention and programming.* Baltimore: Paul H. Brookes.

Chapter 10

MANIPULATIVE ACTIVITIES:
REACH, GRASP, HOLD AND RELEASE

Chapter Objectives: After studying this chapter, the reader will be able to:
1. Differentiate the prehension skills of reach, grasp, hold and release.
2. Assess the child's abilities for reaching, grasping, and releasing.
3. Develop manipulative activities for specific interventions.

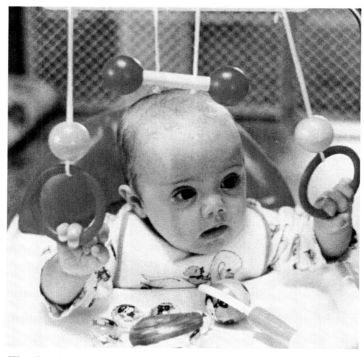

Figure 10.1. The development of reach, grasp, and release is important in acquiring many play skills.

293

This series of activities provides structure to developing fine motor control and eye-hand coordination. The activities are sequenced according to the components of prehension: (a) reaching (adjusting the approach of the hand to an object; (b) grasping (securing the object within the hand); (c) holding (maintaining grasp and manipulating the object); and (d) releasing (letting go of the object). The observational components for assessment of reaching are found in Table 10.1.

Table 10.1. Assessment of Reaching.

Skill	Date Initiated	Date Achieved
1. Focuses on object placed within reach		
2. Brings hands to midline		
3. Reaches for dangling object or toy		
4. Holds object placed in hand		
5. Reaches for object with extended elbow		
6. Extends wrist		
7. Rakes and scoops small objects against palm of hand		
8. Reaches for object bilaterally		
9. Reaches and grasps objects		
10. Reaches for grooming/feeding utensils or other functional items.		
Comments:		

1: Reaching Activities

- Place mobiles or objects in front of child to promote focusing of the eyes (see Figure 10.2).
- Hang pictures, shapes, or favorite objects at appropriate level to promote reaching.
- Use yarn balls, pin wheels, flashlights, colored balls, etc. to promote arm/wrist extension.
- Use mirror play to focus on body awareness.
- Encourage weight bearing on one arm for unilateral reach (see Figure 10.2).
- Have child reach for soap bubbles or balloons.
- Place objects at child's side to encourage reaching across the midline.
- Place objects at a distance that allows the child to explore them using wrist movements.
- During play, place a variety of objects around the child to encourage extended reach.
- Use bolsters, scooter boards, wedges, swinging balls, etc. to encourage distal reach from flexed position.
- Pass objects from hand-to-hand across midline.

The sequence for observational assessment of grasping is found in Table 10.2.

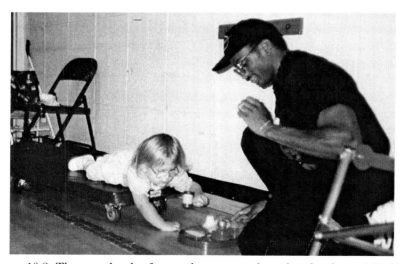

Figure 10.2. The preschooler focuses her eyes and reaches for the activity box.

Table 10.2. Assessment of Grasping.

Skill	Date Initiated	Date Achieved
1. Integration of grasp reflex		
2. Voluntarily grasps an object in palm of hand		
3. Grasps with ulnar palmar prehension (grasps large objects with pinky side of hand and palm)		
4. Grasps with radial palmar prehension - grasps with thumb and 2 fingers		
5. Transfers objects from hand to hand		
6. Thumb opposition of large object (cube)		
7. Grasps small object with interior pincer grasp		
8. Pokes at objects with isolated index finger		
9. Grasps a small object with index finger and thumb (i.e., pincer grasp)		
10. Removes objects from containers		
11. Grasps large crayon/pencil and makes scribble patterns		
12. Maintains grasp on one object while reaching to grasp a second object.		
Comments:		

2: Grasping Activities

Encourage the child to grasp different shaped objects (e.g., doughnut ring, clothespin, blocks, beads, eating utensils) (see Figures 10.3 and 10.4).

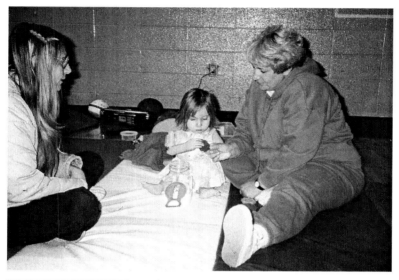

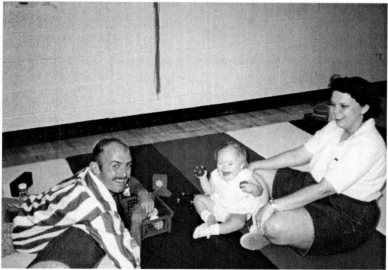

Figures 10.3 and 10.4. The caregiver and movement specialist work together to help child grasp and hold toys.

- Place swinging balls and colored objects in reach of child and encourage him/her to grasp them.
- To increase use of hands encourage manipulation of objects, feeling of textured surfaces, and rolling play dough with rolling pin.
- Encourage weight-bearing on opened hand.
- To extend fingers (to open the hand), have child press on sides of 8" ball or flatten play dough with hands and fingers. Once hand is open, position child over wedge to encourage weight bearing on opened hand.
- Encourage play with push-button toys and dressing dolls/boxes (e.g., zippers, buttons, shoe laces).
- For older children with tight hand and wrist flexors, flex the wrist and apply pressure on the back of the hand so the fingers will extend or release object.
- Encourage performance of age-appropriate game activities.
- Grasp eating utensils.
- Grasp functional utensils (e.g., toothbrush, hairbrush).
- Stack blocks.
- Throw/fling a beanbag or small ball.
- Place various shaped objects in appropriate receptacles.

The observational components for assessment of hold and release are found in Table 10.3.

Table 10.3. Assessment of Hold and Release

Skill	Date Initiated	Date Achieved
1. Holds object		
2. Holds object and releases object voluntarily		
3. Transfers object from hand to hand		
4. Drops object into containers		
5. Stacks blocks		
6. Throws/flings a bean bag or small ball		
7. Places various shaped objects in the appropriate-shaped receptacles		
Comments:		

3: Holding & Releasing Activities

- Demonstrate voluntary release of objects.
- Hold more than one object.
- Hold a container of toys and with the other hand remove the toys.
- Stack and remove rings from tower.
- Stack various size blocks (e.g., 1", 2").
- Peel a banana.
- Play a musical instrument by pressing and releasing keys.
- Place pegs in pegboard.
- Stabilize an object while placing small food (e.g., cereal, raisins) into the container.
- Provide a play area with sand. Let child scoop with one hand while holding container with the other.

- Place lids on pots.
- Use clothespins to grasp objects.
- Screw and unscrew lids on jars.
- String beads, lace shoes.
- Throw balls or beanbag to targets.
- Roll balls to targets.
- Hold and cut forms from paper.
- Turn doorknob and open door.
- Place lids on boxes.
- Fold paper, clothes.
- Unwrap paper from object.

REFERENCES

Brown, S. L., & Donovan, C. M. (1981). *Stimulation activities.* Ann Arbor: University of Michigan.

Brown, S., & Donovan, C. (1989). *Developmental programming for infants and young children—5 volumes.* Ann Arbor: University of Michigan.

Cripe, J., Slentz, K., & Bricker, D. (1993). *Assessment, evaluation, and programming system: Curriculum for birth to three years.* Baltimore: Paul H. Brookes.

Fisher, A. G., Murray, E. A., & Bundy, A. C. (2002). *Sensory integration theory and practice* (2nd ed.). Philadelphia: F.A. Davis.

Frankenburg, W. K., Dodds, J., Archer, P., Bresnick, B., Maschka, P., Edelman, N., & Shapiro, H., (1992). *Denver II.* Denver, CO: Denver Developmental Materials.

Furuno, S., & O'Reilly, K. A., Hosaka, C. M., Inatsuka, T. T, Allman, T. L., & Zeisloft, B. (2005). *HELP activity guide.* Palo Alto, CA: VORT.

Getman, G. N., Kane, E. R., Halgren, M. R., & McKee, G. W. (1968). *Developing learning readiness.* St. Louis, MO: McGraw Hill.

Horvat, M., & Eichstaedt, C. B., (2003). *Developmental/Adapted physical activity: Making ability count* (4th ed.). San Francisco: Benjamin Cummings.

Johnson-Martin, N. M., Jens, K. G. Attermeier, S. M., & Hacker, B. J. (1990). *The Carolina curriculum for preschoolers with special needs.* Baltimore: Paul H. Brookes.

Johnson-Martin, N. M., Jens, K. G., Attermeier, S. M., & Hacker, B. J. (1991). *The Carolina curriculum for infants and toddlers with special needs.* Baltimore: Paul H. Brookes.

Kephart, N. C. (1962). *The slow learner in the classroom.* Columbus, OH: Charles E. Merrill.

Knott, M., & Voss, D. E. (1968). *Proprioceptive neuromuscular facilitation.* New York: Harper & Row.

McCulloch, L. (1983). *A handbook for developing perceptual-motor and sensory skills through body movement.* Austin, TX: Tracor.

Montgomery, P., & Richter, E. (1978). *Sensorimotor integration for developmentally disabled children.* Los Angeles, Western Psychological Services.

Parks, S. (Ed.). (2004). *HELP strands: Curriculum-based developmental assessment.* Palo Alto, CA: VORT.

Parks, S. (2006). *Inside HELP.* Palo Alto, CA: VORT.

Rosato, F. D. (1990). *Fitness and wellness.* St. Paul, MN: West.

Sherrill, C. (2004). *Adapted physical activity, recreation and sport: Crossdisciplinary and lifespan* (6th ed.). New York: McGraw Hill.

Valett, R. E. (1967). *The remediation of learning disability.* Palo Alto, CA: Fearon.

Williamson, G. G. (1987). *Children with spina bifida: Early intervention and programming.* Baltimore: Paul H. Brookes.

GLOSSARY

A

abduction–movement of the extremities away from the midline of the body

abruptio placenta–this condition involves varying degrees of separation of the placenta from the wall of the uterus which interferes with the crucial functions of the placenta

absence seizure–involves unconsciousness for approximately 1–15 seconds suspending mental processes and physical activity

action potential–action that occurs and allows the transmission of information from one neuron to another neuron

adduction–movement of the extremities toward the midline of the body

adenoma sebaceum–tumorous skin glands

adjustment disorders–a disorder which is considered when problems are of a short duration (less than four months) and can be associated with specific environmental occurrence

agnosia–loss of (or diminished) ability to recognize familiar objects

agraphia –loss of handwriting skills

akinesia–loss of movement

alveoli–air pockets of the lungs

amblyopia–refers to problems with the eye's fusional reflexes that interfere with focusing of one eye (lazy eye)

amniotic fluid–the fluid of the womb that serves as a shock absorber for the fetus and provides a temperature-controlled and gravity-free environment

anoxia–loss of oxygen supply to the body's tissues

antagonist–muscles on the opposite side of the joint from the muscles that move the joint or limb. The antagonist muscles relax while the agonist muscles contract and provide the force for movement

apgar–a widely-used method of assessing the infant's health, development, responsivity, and adaptation to extrauterine life

aphasia–loss of language skills

apnea–loss of breathing (usually for 15 to 20 second intervals)

apnea alarm–a monitor that indicates the infant is not breathing or the heart beat is too slow

apraxia/dyspraxia–disorder of motor programming and voluntary movement (without muscle paralysis)

arena assessment–a teaming approach whereby one examiner, the facilitator, administers test items while the other team members observe the child's behavior and score their respective instrument protocols

asperger's syndrome–a form of autism with a child exhibiting a few developmental delays, good communication skills, and more subtle repetitious behaviors

asphyxia–lack of air in lungs which causes suffocation

assessment–any activity designed to elicit accurate and reliable sample behaviors of infants and young children

ataxia–loss of motor coordination and balance

ataxic cerebral palsy–affects a child's ability to coordinate hand movements and to balance during walking due to damage to the cerebellum

athetoid cerebral palsy (also **dyskinesia**)–results in slow, writhing, excessive movements that are accentuated during voluntary movement attempts, fluctuations in muscle tone, and difficulty with coordination of posture and locomotion due to damage to the extrapyramidal tract of the brain

athetosis–excessive random movements caused by damage to the extrapyramidal system of the central nervous system

atonic seizure–momentary loss of muscle tone which may cause the individual to sag or collapse

attachment deprivation–may be the result of the child receiving inadequate physical, psychological, and emotional care

auditory discrimination–the ability to distinguish changes in volume intensity, pitch/frequency, rhythm, or other tonal qualities of sound

autism spectrum disorder–includes the three common disorders of: Autism, Asperger's Disorder and Pervasive Developmental Disorder Not Otherwise Specified; as well as semantic pragmatic communication disorder, nonverbal learning disabilities, high functioning autism, heperlexia and some aspects of ADHD

autonomic hyperreflexia (dysreflexia)–an uninhibited reflex response to a stimulus

autonomic nervous system–division of the nervous system which governs the balance of the internal organs of the body

autosomal dominant disorder–caused by an alteration in a single gene along one of the autosomes

autosomal recessive disorder–occurs with 25% statistical risk when both parents are carriers of the altered gene

autosomes–the 22 pair of chromosomes combined from the father and mother but not the X and Y chromosome termed the sex chromosome

axon–a single long process of a neuron responsible for transmission of sensory data to a dendrite of another neuron

B
bacterial meningitis–pathological germs which infect the membranes surrounding the brain

balance–postural control

barotrauma–trauma associated with high inflation pressures which may lead to bronchopulmonary dysplasia

basal ganglia–a group of nuclei that regulate and modulate cortical information from almost every area of the cerebral hemispheres

bilateral movements–movements of both sides of the body or the upper and lower parts of the body

bilirubin–a yellow-orange pigment which normally circulates in plasma and is metabolized by liver cells

bradycardia–slow heart beat of less than 60 beats per minute

brain stem–an upward extension of the spinal cord subdivided into a stem-like portion comprising the medulla, pons, and midbrain

breech position–the newborn's buttocks precede the head during delivery

bronchopulmonary dysplasia–is a chronic lung disease caused by respiratory distress of infants related to oxygen toxicity or barotrauma, which is characterized by interstitial fibrosis and bronchiolar metaplasia (abnormal tissue changes); requires mechanical ventilation and supplemental oxygen

C
cataract–opacity (not clear, not transparent) of the eye caused by injury, exposure to great heat or radiation, or an inherited factor

cephalocaudal development–human motor development occurs from the head downward to the feet

cerebellum–the second largest portion of the brain; regulates muscular coordination for balance and integrates postural and equilibrium reactions; provides for the automatic phase of movements that no longer require conscious thought

cerebral aqueduct–connects the third and fourth ventricles located in the midbrain

cerebral palsy–a nonprogressive neuromuscular condition resulting from damage to the central nervous system during the early stages of development

cerebrum (cerebral) cortex–the largest portion of the human brain and the main center for voluntary movement, learning, perception, memory, and communication

chorioretinitis–inflammation of the choroid (area between the sclera and retina) and the retina

chromosome—a chain of deoxyribonucleic acid which transmits genetic information

cleft lip and palate—congenital split of the lip or roof of the mouth

contracture—a permanent shortening of muscles, tendons, or scar tissues which results in an inability to stretch or extend the muscle

contraindicated position—a position that would not be recommended for the child to experience optimal development

contralateral movements—movements on one side of the body may affect the opposite side of the body

convergent assessment—a process that incorporates information from various assessments, sources, occasions, and settings to describe the child's developmental status

corpus callosum—connects the right and left cerebral hemispheres

cranial nerves—12 pair of nerves that are attached to the brain and pass through the openings of the skull

criterion test—comparison of development or skill to a predetermined criteria

cross-disciplinary team—individuals representing selected disciplines of study who collaborate professionally to determine specific interventions

crosslateral movements—movements that cross the midline of the body

curriculum-based assessment—a form of skill appraisal that determines the child's achievement and instructional needs along a continuum of objectives within course content

cytomegalovirus (CMV)—a herpes virus that may be passed across the placenta in utero or contracted as the newborn ascends through the birth canal

D

deoxyribonucleic acid (DNA)—the basic structure of genes

dendrite—an extension of the neuron responsible for receiving sensory information from the outside world

development—functional changes which lead to compensation by the individual throughout the lifespan

developmental delay—a slowing in the onset of expected developmental outcomes or milestones

diplopia—the child perceives there are two images of an object; double vision

distal—moving further away from a certain point

dorsal roots—sensory nerve fibers of a spinal nerve

dorsiflexion—upward movement of the foot or hand

Down syndrome—a genetic abnormality caused by one of three types of chromosomal defects: nondisjunction, translocation, and mosaicism; instead of the normal 46 chromosomes (23 pair); individuals with Down syndrome have an extra 21st chromosome due to failure of the 21st chromosome pair to separate

duration–how long an exercise is performed

dysarthria–impaired motor control of all the muscles for producing speech and articulating words due to damage to the central or peripheral nervous system

dyskinesia–impairment of voluntary movements resulting in fragmented or jerking motion in fine motor muscle groups

dysmetria–impaired ability to estimate distance in muscular action resulting in an inability to position the limbs accurately with respect to another object

dysmorphologist–someone who studies genetics

dysphagia–difficulty swallowing

E

eating disorders–behaviors such as unhealthy attitude toward eating, hoarding of food, reduction in body weight, and nutritional deficiencies

ecological assessment–includes the interactions between the individual and all aspects of his or her respective environment

encephalitis–acute or chronic infections of the brain

equilibrium or tilting reactions–compensatory movements which allow the child to adjust posture and maintain stability while in the prone, supine, sitting, quadruped, or standing positions

excitation–increasing muscle tension

extension–straightening of the extremities

extrapyramidal system–a major pathway for movement related to movements of automatic control and postural reactions

extremely low birth weight–refers to an infant who is born weighing less than 750 grams (1 lb. 10 oz.)

extremity–the arm or leg

F

facia dysmorphism–abnormal facial formation during early fetal development

failure-to-thrive–developmental and physical retardation in children due to factors such as physical illness or maternal deprivation

febrile seizures–tonic-clonic seizures that are a result of high fevers; they typically terminate when fever disappears

feedback–the return of sensory information to its source so the output may be modified or improved

fetal alcohol syndrome–abnormalities that result from exposure to alcohol during gestation; the most common environmental cause of mental retardation in the developed countries

fetal hydantoin syndrome–(also known as **fetal dilantin syndrome**)–abnormalities that result from teratogenic effects of anticonvulsant drugs

flaccidity–low muscle tone; the muscle may feel soft or mushy; little resistance to stretching

flexion–bending of the extremities

focal-motor seizure–one of the most common partial seizures, sometimes referred to as a Jacksonian march. Muscle twitching begins in one part of the body and may move to include other body parts

fragile X syndrome–also know as Martin-Bell syndrome and Marker X syndrome; X-linked inherited syndrome

frequency–how often an exercise is performed

G

gametes–sex cells

gametic meiotic reduction division–one of each pair of autosomes and one of the sex chromosomes are distributed randomly to each daughter cell

gastroesophageal reflux–reflux of the stomach and duodenal contents into the espohagus; the child may also experience heartburn and regurgitation; the condition is chronic and potentially life-threatening

gastroschisis–a congenital defect of the abdominal wall which typically appears to be to the right of the umbilical cord; the intestine is thickened, shortened and usually malrotated; the bowel is extruded and may include the stomach

gastrostomy–a surgical procedure that is performed when infants are not able to suck or swallow enough nutrients for adequate and proper oral nutrition; a tube is placed directly into the stomach of the baby for feeding and is kept in place by a special dressing

gene–a part of a chromosome which makes up some portions of DNA; heredity is influenced by the genes an offspring receives from the parents; the daily functions and reproduction of all cells are controlled by the genes

geneticist–someone who specialized in the study of heredity

growth–quantitative biological and structural changes of the physical size of the child

H

handling–hands-on moving of the child from one place to another

hepatitis B virus (serum hepatitis)–a virus, transmitted through body *flu-*

ids, which causes inflammation of the liver and can remain in body fluids for years or even a lifetime

herpes–an aggressive virus that may appear in the newborn as a localized infection, but may spread to a systemic disease

holding–maintaining grasp to manipulate an object

human immunodeficiency virus (HIV)–virus that infects the human body; as the infection worsens, the disease AIDS may result.

hydrocephalus–a complication occurring from hemorrhage within the ventricular system, interruption of circulation, or reabsorption of cerebral spinal fluid causing a back-up of fluid, increased intracranial pressure, and expansion of the ventricles

hymonymous hemianopsia–loss of the same part of the visual field in both eyes

hyperactive gag reflex–an overactive or extremely sensitive gag reflex

hyperbilirubinemia–results from too much bilirubin in the blood as a result of liver or biliary tract dysfunction or increased destruction of red blood cells

hypertonia–excessive, spastic, or increased muscle tone

hypothalamus–responsible for regulation and integration of autonomic nervous system responses, temperature control, water balance, food intake and gastric secretions, heart rate, and expression of emotions

hypothyroidism–an autosomal recessive metabolic disorder in which there is a disorder of thyroid hormone production causing the infant to be small, hypotonic, and severely mentally retarded

hypotonia–weak, floppy, or decreased tone

hypoxia–reduced or low oxygen supply to tissues

hypoxia ischemic encephalopathy–a lack of oxygen and inadequate blood supply may cause acute or chronic infections of the brain and result in seizures, abnormal muscle tone and reflexes, respiratory distress, and signs of neurological dysfunction

I

inhibition–the restraining of an activity or process

intensity–degree of exerted effort to perform an exercise, during each bout of exercise

interdisciplinary teams–professionals who develop collaborative goals and individual service plans for young children

intersensory integration–the ability to simultaneously use information from several sensory systems, enabling adaptation to the environment and problem solving

intersensory modality stimulation–receiving information into the central nervous system (brain and spinal cord) from several sensory modalities that result in excitatory or inhibitory responses

intrauterine growth retardation–results when an fetus' intrauterine growth has been slowed or diminished causing the baby to be small for gestational age

intraventricular hemorrhage–an extremely serious and common neurological disorder of premature infants whereby grades or levels are characterized by hemorrhage or bleeding and the areas of the brain tissue that are affected

ipsilateral–refers to the same side of the body

ischemia–inadequate blood supply

J

Jacksonian seizure (focal-motor seizure)–results in muscular twitching which begins in one area of the body and may spread to the entire body

jaundice–high blood bilirubin levels in the infant may result in yellow coloration to the skin

joint laxity–an unusual amount of mobility/range of motion in joints

judgment-based assessment–formal process of collecting, structuring, and quantifying ideas and observations of professionals and caregivers about child environmental characteristics

K

karotyping–a process through which diagnosis of abnormality is completed

kernicterus–a clinical syndrome of abnormalities that result from hyperbilirubinemia

kinesthetic–a sensory modality that provides information about position of one's limbs in space, thus assisting in controlling and coordinating movement; receptors are proprioceptors located in muscles, tendons, and joints

L

locomotor–moving from one place to another, changing location of one's body, e.g., creeping, walking, running

low birth weight–refers to an infant who is born weighing less than 2,500 grams (5 pounds)

lower motor neuron–spinal cord lesions that cause flaccid muscle tone

M

maturation–qualitative changes that occur as a function of time and age

meconium–an accumulation of feces in the bowel of the fetus

meconium aspiration–inhalation of feces into lung passages with first respiratory efforts

medulla oblongata–an upper extension of the spinal cord as it enters the brain

metacarpals–the bones between the wrist and the fingers

microcephaly–an unusually small head circumference defined by decreases in size of two standard deviations below the mean

midbrain–the portion of the brain between the pons and the cerebral hemispheres composed of the superior and inferior colliculi

midline–arbitrary line down the center of the body from head to toe that distinguishes the left and right sides of the body

mitosis–each replicated chromosome is pulled apart longitudinally at the centromere so that each daughter cell has identical chromosome complements (46 chromosomes)

mixed cerebral palsy–refers to the presence of more than one type of cerebral palsy without any one type being dominant

mobility–active movement

mode–method or type of exercise

motor development–changes of movement behavior across the lifespan including growth, development, and maturation

motor neurons–convey messages from the central nervous system to the muscles resulting in a reflex, reaction, or motor skill; also referred to as efferent neurons

multidisciplinary team–professionals who perform assessments independent of one another, have very little collaboration, and view their specific roles as separate from the other disciplines

muscle tone–contractile tension and readiness of muscles to perform movement

muscular endurance–the ability of muscles to sustain repeated contractions

myelin–the innermost fatty covering of nerve fibers

myelination–the process of forming a white protein insulating covering of nerve fiber pathways within the central nervous system

myoclonic seizure–brief, sudden violent contractions that may occur in one body part or in the entire body

N

necrotizing entercolitis (NEC)–a serious condition that affects the bowel wall in many preterm infants; associated with severe hypoxic or anoxic insult to bowel wall causing necrosis

Neonatal Intensive Care Unit (NICU)–a critical care unit of a level III hospital prepared for taking care of mother and infant at high risk for survival

nerve cell (also **neuron**)–the functional unit of the nervous system

nonlocomotor–moving body parts through space, but not moving one's body to another place in the invironment. Body movements in place, e.g., twisting, bending, turning

nonviable—incapable of living

norm-referenced—assessment that compares an individual's performance in relationship to others who are similar; it determines how an individual compares to a normative group.

nuchal rigidity—reflex spasm of the neck extensor muscles; results in resistance to cervical flexion

nystagimus—an involuntary rapid movement of the eyeball.

O

obturator—a cover that is inserted in the opening of a new tracheostomy tube to serve as a guide for easy insertion

orthoptic vision—vision affected by the six external muscles which control movement of the eyeball

orthotics—biomedical equipment used to protect, train, or restore an existing body segment

P

palpebral fissures—longitudinal opening between eyelids

parachute reactions—protective extension movements that occur when the child starts to fall or lose his balance

paresis—incomplete paralysis: weakness

patent ductus arteriosis (PDA)—failure of the fetal ductus ateriosis to completely close after birth

perceptual-motor—acquiring and using information gained through the integrated processes of sensation and perception to guide movement

perinatal asphyxia—a lack of oxygen and excess carbon dioxide in the newborn's blood that occurs during the birth process and results in loss of consciousness

perinatal trauma—trauma that occurs shortly before, during or after birth

peripheral nervous system—system outside of the spinal cord and brain; consist of 31 pair of spinal nerves and 12 pair of cranial nerves

periventricular leukomalacia—resulting from premature birth, this condition leads to hemorrhage in the ventricles of the brain

perseveration—persistent involuntary repetition of a verbal or motor response beyond presence of stimulus

pervasive developmental disorder (PDD)—communication disorders that include: Autistic disorder, Rett's Disorder, Childhood Disintegrative Disorder, Asperger's Disorder, and PDD Not Otherwise Specified

petechiae—bleeding spots

phasic tone—a rapid contraction in response to a high degree of stretch

phenylketonuria (PKU)—an inherited autosomal recessive inborn error of amino acid metabolism whereby the child's system does not produce a necessary liver enzyme therefore allowing the amino acid, phenylalanine, to build up in the blood stream until it becomes toxic

pituitary–pertaining to the pituitary (endocrine) gland at the base of the brain

placenta–the organ that joins mother and child during pregnancy and provides endocrine secretion and exchange of blood-borne substances and nutrients

placenta previa–fertilized egg is introduced in the bottom of the uterus instead of the top of the uterus causing the placenta to implant and cover the opening of the cervix

plantar flexion–downward movement of foot or hand

pons–forms a "bridge of fibers" connecting the medulla to the cerebellum

positioning–static movement of the child

postural reaction–automatic responses that assist in maintaining equilibrium and balance

postural tone–a prolonged contraction in response to a low-intensity stretch

posturing–abnormal positioning of body or body parts

Prader-Willi syndrome–a result of partial deletion of chromosome 15; abnormalities include mild to moderate mental retardation, an obsession for eating, and subsequent serious obesity and hypotonia

prehension–grasp involving opposition of thumb and fingers

premature labor–contractions of uterus and cervical dilation prior to 37 weeks of gestation

prematurity–birth prior to 37 weeks gestation; the infant weighs less than 2,500 grams

primitive reflexes–typical, involuntary flexor and extensor movements that occur during the first year of life and must be inhibited or integrated by the central nervous system

progressive interactive assessment–a multicomponent, concentrated, progressive process which emphasizes the quality of services to be provided to the child and family

prone–lying on the stomach

proprioception–sensing (or knowing) the movement and position of the body parts in relation to each other and to gravity

prosthetics–biomedical equipment used to replace body parts

proximal–near to a point of reference

proximodistal development–muscular movements near the midline of the body become more refined before those more distal to the body

psychophysiological response to stress–involuntary interaction of psychological (mind) and physiological (body) processes in response to non-specific demands

psychomotor seizure–involves blinking, lip smacking, facial grimacing, groaning, chewing, or other automatic actions which occur for 30 seconds to 5 minutes

ptosis–drooping of the upper eyelid

pyramidal system–one of the major motor pathways for movement control that stimulates or initiates muscular activity and is responsible for precise movements necessary for fine and skillful coordination

R

range of motion–movement of joints of the body in all planes

reaching–adjusting the approach of one's hand to an object

reactions–automatic movements that replace the primitive reflexes with unique functions necessary for the development of balance

reciprocal innervation–the interaction of muscles contracting while the opposite muscles stretch or relax allowing for freedom of movement of bones and joints

reflex arc–the completion of a neural circuit; composed of a receptor, afferent input neuron, connecting or internuncial neuron, and efferent output neuron, and a muscle or organ that produces activity

releasing–letting go of an object

repetitions–the number of times a muscle is required to contract during a specific exercise

respiratory distress syndrome–results from lung immaturity and absence of necessary surfactant which prevents the lungs from collapsing during normal breathing in premature infants

rest–required of muscle to prevent fatigue

reticular activating system–comprised of the medulla, pons, and midbrain, the RAS serves to screen incoming sensory stimulation inhibiting some sensory input and processing other information

retinitis–inflammation of the retina

retinopathy of prematurity (ROP)–a disorder that interrupts the vascularization of the maturing retina; caused by low birth weight, gestation age, and too much oxygen

retrolental fibroplasia–complete visual impairment due to prolonged and high oxygen concentrations commonly referred to as ROP

righting reactions–automatic movements that assist with the alignment of the head and the trunk with each other and help to develop balance

rigid cerebral palsy–results in severely limited movement due to hypertonicity of flexor and extensor muscles that result from damage to the extrapyramidal tract; the most severe type of cerebral palsy

rubella (German measles)–an infection which may result in abnormal physical anomalies or developmental disabilities in the newborn if contracted by the mother during the first four months of pregnancy

S

screening–assessment to determine if a more in-depth evaluation is needed

segmental innervation–involves an area of the skin supplied by dendrites from one dorsal root ganglia projecting into one spinal cord segment and one ventral root of the spinal cord and the underlying muscles or portions of muscle

seizure (convulsions)–involuntary motor activity that results from an electrical-chemical imbalance in the regulatory center of the brain

sensation–the reception of internal and external stimuli for which the primary purpose is to provide information about the functioning of the body

spina bifida meningocele–meninges (spinal cord covering) protrude in the sac outside the body, but cord and nerves are not displaced outside the body. Surgical correction is needed.

spinal bifida myelomeningocele (MM)–the most severe form of spina bifida where spinal cord and nerve roots fill a sac outside the body. Surgical correction is needed and paralysis is frequent.

spina bifida occulta–the mildest form of spina bifida where there is some abnormality of development but no protrusion of the cord or its membrane. The condition is concealed under the skin and paralysis or muscle weakness does not occur. Occulta is not often diagnosed until later in life when other back problems occur and x-rays are taken.

sensory neurons–relay information from the end receptors (skin, muscles, tendons, joints, organs) to the spinal cord and brain; also referred to as afferent neurons

sepsis–any viral, bacterial, or parasitic infection that the child acquires shortly after birth

sets–the number of times an exercise should be repeated

sex chromosome–the 23rd pair of chromosomes determines the child's gender

short palpebral fissures–eye slits which cause eyes to appear to be wide-set

small for gestational age–refers to birth weight less than the third percentile

somatosensory processing–the combination of input from the tactile sensory modality and proprioceptive sensation

spastic cerebral palsy–occurs as a result of damage to the pyramidal tract of the brain; there is increased motor neuronal excitability and enhanced stretch–evoked synaptic excitation of motor neurons, muscle tightening, and hypertonia; the most common type of cerebral palsy

spasticity–excessive flexor or extensor contraction; increased muscle tone;

easy excitability and impairment of volitional ability to relax

spatial relations–the child may have difficulty perceiving the position or relationship of two or more objects

spina bifida–a congenital defect involving failure of part of the spine and spinal cord to close

stability–holding strategies

standardized test–provide normative data which allow comparisons between children

stoma–an opening for drainage or tube insertion

strabismus–refers to eye muscles that are not in balance causing a problem with visual alignment of the eyes (i.e., crossed-eyes)

strength–the force exerted by muscles in a single contraction

supine–the backlying position

surfactant–a lubricant that facilitates adequate lung expansion

synapse–site of communication between neurons through the exchange of a chemical message or neurotransmitter

syndactyly–webbing of the fingers or toes

syphilis–a disease caused by a microorganism, Treponema palladium, that is passed from mother to newborn through the placenta, or as the baby moves through the birth canal

T

tactile defensiveness–a negative response to certain tactile stimuli

tactile discrimination–the ability to recognize, perceive and organize information involving touch

tactile integration–the differentiation among the sensory stimuli located in the skin (light touch, pressure, pain, and temperature)

thalamus–organizes and integrates sensory impulses and responds to the emotions of fear, rage, and pleasant or unpleasant sensations

therapeutic riding–horseback riding activities designed for individuals with disabilities that provide relaxation of muscles, improvement of balance and posture, socialization, concentration, self-esteem, and discipline

theory–a set of ideas formulated by principles

tonic-clonic seizure–during the tonic phase of this type of seizure, the body stiffens in rigid muscular contraction and consciousness is lost; during the clonic phase, jerking, uncontrolled body movements occur, and respiration and swallowing is interrupted

TORCH–an acronym that reflects the commonly encountered diseases toxoplasmosis, rubella, cytomegalovirus, herpes, and syphilis which cause some similar malformations in the fetus

toxoplasmosis–an infection that results from a parasite, toxoplasma protozoan, which is transmitted from the mother to the fetus

tracheostomy–an opening in the trachea or windpipe that the infant will breathe through instead of the nose and mouth; a short piece of plastic is surgically placed in the hole in the windpipe and does not connect to the lungs

traction response–the most often used method of assessing postural tone in a young child; demonstrated by pulling the child by the arms to sitting and noting the amount of head lag and elbow flexion

transactional assessment–involves observation and interview to assess the physical environment and interactions between the child, caregiver, and professional

transdisciplinary teams–professionals who encourage a role sharing approach to intervention whereby one or two team members are responsible for the implementation of actual intervention goals

tremor cerebral palsy–uncontrolled involuntary and rhythmic movements due to damage to the cerebellum or basal ganglia

tuberous sclerosis–an autosomal dominant or sporadic disorder which results in seizures, mental retardation, adenoma sebaceum, calcium deposits in the brain, malignancies, hydrocephalus and tumors of the heart; the child has an unusual "butterfly" rash on the face

Turner syndrome–also known as XO syndrome, this syndrome is found only in females and is a sex chromosome abnormality that occurs when one of the two X chromosomes is absent or partially absent

U

umbilical cord–contains all nutrients and oxygenated blood from the *fetus* side of the placenta and connects to the fetus

unilateral movements–movements occurring on one side of the body

upper motor neuron (UMN)–neurons in the cerebral cortex that conduct impulses from the motor cortex to motor nuclei of the cerebral nerves or to the ventral gray columns of the spinal cord

V

ventral roots–motor nerve fibers of a spinal nerve

ventriculo-peritoneal shunt–drains cerebral spinal fluid from the brain to the abdominal cavity preventing major developmental delays from hydrocephalus

very low birth weight–refers to an infant who is born weighing less than 1,500 grams (3 lbs. 5 oz.)

vestibular modality–the sensory system which is responsible for the development of equilibrium and balance

visual acuity–refers to refractive vision or the amount of light rays bending and reaching the visual receptors (rods and cones)

visual figure-ground perception–the ability to identify and focus on relevant object(s) in one's visual field and distinguish them or pick them out from the background

visual motor control–the ability to coordinate eye movements to allow for fixation, tracking of moving objects, figure-ground perception, and discrimination of forms, shapes and sizes

visual motor discrimination–the ability to discriminate between objects that differ in external form, size, color, texture, number, or position in space

X

X-linked dominant disorders–mutation of the X chromosome or XX in females

X-linked recessive disorders–mutation of the XY chromosome in males who have no normal gene to lessen the impact; usually results in severe or lethal effects

AUTHOR INDEX

319

SUBJECT INDEX

ABOUT THE AUTHORS

Joe E. Cowden, Ph.D.

Doctor Cowden has been a professor of adapted physical education and motor development at The University of New Orleans for the past 26 years. She also served as director of the UNO Adapted Physical Education and Motor Development Clinic. In addition, she served as project director of three federally funded training grants, Project IMPACT with Bobby Eason (Imitable Physical Activity Curriculum Theory), Project PAMD (Pediatric Adapted Motor Development, and Project PAPE (Pediatric Adapted Physical Education). She created and developed Project GUMBO (Louisiana Games Uniting Mind and Body) which is coordinated by the Louisiana State Department of Education. The track and field games are for children who have physical disabilities with high cognitive abilities. Doctor Cowden has brought in over $1.5 million into The University of New Orleans through numerous grants and contracts.

Doctor Cowden served as Project Director of the Third International Symposium on Adapted Physical Activity hosted by The University of New Orleans in 1980 which was the beginning of her tenure at The University of New Orleans. Most recently in 2000, Doctor Cowden served as the Symposium Director of the Fifth North American Federation of Adapted Physical Activity Symposium at the Monteleone Hotel in New Orleans. Due to the visit of the storm named Katrina, The University of New Orleans eliminated the Department of Human Performance and Health Promotion, and Doctor Cowden took early retirement.

Specializing in assessment and program development for infants and children and their families for 26 years at The University of New Orleans Adapted Motor Development Clinic was very rewarding. Undergraduate, graduate students and teachers who were working on their 21-hour adapted physical education certification served as teachers for the individualized, instructional program for the infants and young children. Approximately 95 percent of the certified adapted physical education teachers of the Greater New Orleans area completed their certification program and masters degrees with Doctor Cowden from 1980–2006.

Doctor Cowden served on the editorial board of the *Adapted Physical Activity Quarterly* from 1997 to 2005. She also serves as manuscript and abstract reviewer for several national journals. She has made over 100 presentations throughout the United States, Canada, and Spain. In addition, she has published extensively with over 75 book chapters or publications in national and state journals including the

Adapted Physical Activity Quarterly and *Journal of Health and Physical Education* with the most recent being the second revision of this book.

Doctor Cowden completed her baccalaureate degree from Midwestern State University, Wichita Falls, TX, master of arts degree from Sam Houston State University, Huntsville, TX and the doctor of philosophy degree from Texas Woman's University, Denton, TX, under the direction of Doctors Claudine Sherrill and Jane Mott.

Carol C. Torrey, Ph.D.

Carol Torrey is currently employed as a Special Education Program Coordinator in the Jefferson Parish Public School System, Marrero, Louisiana. Doctor Torrey coordinates the Adapted Physical Education program and supervises 30 full-time adapted physical education teachers that provide services to students with identified motor impairments. The Adapted Physical Education Program is one of the largest in the state of Louisiana and has included innovative motor, fitness, and recreational programs for children between the ages of 3 and 22 years. Prior to returning to the public schools, Doctor Torrey was an Associate Professor in the Department of Teaching and Learning at Southeastern Louisiana University, Hammond, Louisiana. Her major emphasis was the development and expansion of the Early Childhood Special Education Program (special education for children birth to 5 years) and included teaching graduate-level students, involvement in state and community early intervention projects, research in the field of early intervention and supervising student internships in centers for infants, toddlers, and preschoolers. For the past 10 years, she has served on the Board of Directors for the Regina Coeli Child Development Center, which includes 13 Head Start and Early Head Start programs in six parishes (counties) and Families Helping Families, a family advocacy program for families with individuals with disabilities. She has published and presented at professional conferences in the areas of adapted physical education, special education, behavioral issues, and early intervention. Doctor Torrey earned a baccalaureate degree in Health and Physical Education from The University of New Orleans. Her doctor of philosophy was earned from the Department of Special Education and Habilitative Services from The University of New Orleans under supervision of Doctors Jo E. Cowden and David Sexton.

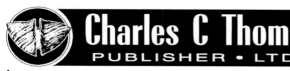

Charles C Thomas
PUBLISHER • LTD.

P.O. Box 19265
Springfield, IL 62794-9265

• Cowden, Jo E. & Carol C. Torrey—**MOTOR DEVELOPMENT AND MOVEMENT ACTIVITIES FOR PRESCHOOLERS AND INFANTS WITH DELAYS: A Multisensory Approach for Professionals and Families. (2nd Ed.)** '07, 308 pp. (7 x 10), 195 il., 13 tables.

Thoroughly revised and updated, this second edition continues to present a theoretical and practical approach to motor development and adapted physical activity programs for infants and toddlers with disabilities. Written from a broad perspective, the authors use easy-to-understand language so that families, caregivers, and students may provide instruction utilizing the ecological dynamics of the home environment. Chapter topics include: motor development, organization of the nervous system, muscle tone, medical and biological considerations, prematurity and low birth weight, assessment, principles of intervention, and progressive interactive facilitation. The book explains the principles of motor development theories and relates them to practical intervention, and answers questions related to positioning, lifting, carrying, and feeding of young children. In addition, practical suggestions and activities for families and professionals to enhance sensory motor development of the young child during structured motor intervention and throughout the day are given. Generously illustrated, this comprehensive book is an excellent resource for training adapted physical educators, early interventionists, and caregivers in pediatric motor development. It will also serve as a reference for individuals developing motor programs for older children, particularly children with severe delays.

• Crandell, John M. Jr. & Lee W. Robinson—**LIVING WITH LOW VISION AND BLINDNESS: Guidelines That Help Professionals and Individuals Understand Vision Impairments.** '07, 222 pp. (7 x 10), 14 il.

• Hargis, Charles H.—**ENGLISH SYNTAX: An Outline for Teachers of English Language Learners. (3rd Ed.)** '07, 246 pp. (7 x 10), 6 tables, 6 il.

• Bryan, Willie V.—**MULTICULTURAL ASPECTS OF DISABILITIES: A Guide to Understanding and Assisting Minorities in the Rehabilitation Process. (2nd Ed.)** '07, 348 pp. (7 x 10), $69.95, hard, $49.95, paper.

• Martin, E. Davis, Jr.—**PRINCIPLES AND PRACTICES OF CASE MANAGEMENT IN REHABILITATION COUNSELING. (2nd Ed.)** '07, 380 pp. (7 x 10), 7 il., 2 tables, $69.95, hard, $49.95, paper.

• Mithaug, Dennis E., Deirdre K. Mithaug, Martin Agran, James E. Martin, & Michael L. Wehmeyer—**SELF-INSTRUCTION PEDAGOGY: How to Teach Self-Determined Learning.** '07, 242 pp. (8 x 10), 57 il., 87 tables, $64.95, hard, $44.95, paper.

• Drummond, Sakina S.—**NEUROGENIC COMMUNICATION DISORDERS: Aphasia and Cognitive-Communication Disorders.** '06, 246 pp. (7 x 10), 25 il., 17 tables, $55.95, hard, $35.95, paper.

• Soby, Jeanette M.—**PRENATAL EXPOSURE TO DRUGS/ALCOHOL: Character- and Educational Implications of Fetal Alcohol Syndrome and Cocaine/Polydrug Effects. (2nd Ed.)** '06, 188 pp. (7 x 10), 7 il., 21 tables, $44.95, hard, $28.95, paper.

• Craig, Robert J.—**ASSESSING SUBSTANCE ABUSERS WITH THE MILLON CLINICAL MULTIAXIAL INVENTORY (MCMI).** '05, 164 pp. (7 x 10), 16 il., 15 tables, $46.95, hard, $26.95, paper.

• Kass, Corrine E. & Cleborne D. Maddux—**A HUMAN DEVELOPMENT VIEW OF LEARNING DISABILITIES: From Theory to Practice. (2nd Ed.)** '05, 252 pp. (7 x 10), 5 tables, $55.95, hard, $35.95, paper.

• Hoffman, Cheryl M.—**COMPREHENSIVE REFERENCE MANUAL FOR SIGNERS AND INTERPRETERS. (5th Ed.)** '03, 344 pp. (8 1/2 x 11), $59.95, spiral (paper).

• Pollack, Doreen, Donald Goldberg & Nancy Coleffe-Schenck—**EDUCATIONAL AUDIOLOGY FOR THE LIMITED-HEARING INFANT AND PRESCHOOLER: An Auditory-Verbal Program. (3rd Ed.)** '97, 410 pp. (7 x 10), 46 il., 18 tables, $100.95, cloth, $76.95, paper.

• Laban, Richard J.—**CHEMICAL DEPENDENCY TREATMENT PLANNING HANDBOOK.** '97, 174 pp. (8 1/2 x 11), $35.95, spiral (paper).

• Stryker, Stephanie—**SPEECH AFTER STROKE: A Manual for the Speech-Language Pathologist and the Family Member. (2nd Ed.)** '81, 442 pp., 179 il., $57.95, spiral (paper).

 easy ways to order!

PHONE:
1-800-258-8980
or (217) 789-8980

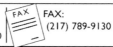 FAX:
(217) 789-9130

EMAIL:
books@ccthomas.com
Web: www.ccthomas.com

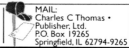 MAIL:
Charles C Thomas •
Publisher, Ltd.
P.O. Box 19265
Springfield, IL 62794-9265

Complete catalog available at ccthomas.com • books@ccthomas.com

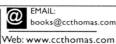

Books sent on approval • Shipping charges: $7.75 min. U.S. / Outside U.S., actual shipping fees will be charged • Prices subject to change without notice
Savings include all titles shown here and on our web site. For a limited time only.